Do you have two or more of these symptoms?

- High blood pressure
- High blood cholesterol levels
- Obesity
- Increased thirst and urination
- Fluctuating changes in vision
- Unexplained weight loss
- Fatigue
- Wounds that do not heal
- Infertility (in women)

If so, you could be suffering from Syndrome X.

CHECK WITH YOUR DOCTOR FOR A COMPLETE DIAGNOSIS

SYNDROME X

MANAGING INSULIN RESISTANCE

DEBORAH S. ROMAINE AND JENNIFER B. MARKS, M.D.

WITH A FOREWORD BY GLENN S. ROTHFELD, M.D.

Produced by Amaranth

HarperTorch

An Imprint of HarperCollins*Publishers*

SYNDROME X is not a substitute for sound medical advice. The ideas, procedures, and suggestions in this book are intended to supplement, not replace, the advice of a trained medical professional. All matters regarding your health require medical supervision. Consult your physician before adopting the suggestions in this book, as well as about any condition that may require diagnosis or medical attention. The authors, book producer, and publisher disclaim any liability arising directly or indirectly from the use of this book.

❦

HARPERTORCH
An Imprint of HarperCollins*Publishers*
10 East 53rd Street
New York, New York 10022-5299

Copyright © 2000 by Amaranth
ISBN: 0-380-81444-7

First HarperTorch paperback printing: December 2000

HarperCollins®, HarperTorch™, and ❦ ™ are trademarks of Harper-Collins Publishers Inc.

Printed in the United States of America

Visit HarperTorch on the World Wide Web at www.harpercollins.com

10 9 8 7 6 5 4 3 2 1

~

Contents

Foreword

Insulin was no mystery when I learned about it in medical school 28 years ago. Insulin lowered glucose (sugar) in the bloodstream, and without it glucose built up and spilled into the urine. Diabetics were low in insulin; we gave insulin for type 1 diabetics, which we called juvenile-onset diabetics and glucose-lowering drugs for type 2 diabetics, called adult-onset diabetics. Diabetics had increased hardening of the arteries, increased circulatory and vision problems, decreased healing, and decreased life expectancy. We spent a lot of time controlling blood sugar levels, but we didn't pay much attention to insulin itself.

We were, of course, aware that adult-onset diabetics tended to be obese. Insulin levels in these people were actually elevated, and their cells were relatively resistant to insulin. When these diabetics lost weight, their blood sugar levels became more normal, and their insulin levels moved toward normal as well. We also were painfully aware of how difficult it was for adult-onset diabetics to lose weight, and so we didn't have many successful strategies to help them.

All this has changed in the past fifteen years, since Dr. George Reaven and his colleagues at the Stanford University School of Medicine coined the term *syndrome X* to describe the cluster of conditions associated with insulin resistance. These conditions occur in as many as 25% of the population, according to some estimates. The conditions include elevation of triglycerides and LDL cholesterol, the "bad" cholesterol. Blood pressures tend to be elevated. Menstrual irregularities, particularly a condition known as polycystic ovaries, are more common. And even the body shape (so-called "apple" shape) is different.

Many of these people go on to develop type 2 diabetes. Many others have symptoms of blood sugar fluctuations and sugar cravings. All people with syndrome X have increased risk of strokes, heart attacks, and the organ damage associated with diabetes.

Deborah S. Romaine and Dr. Jennifer B. Marks have written a very readable and thorough book describing syndrome X and its relationship to diabetes. They have also included some very practical information on the dietary and lifestyle management of syndrome X. This is a critical part of the book as syndrome X is, if nothing else, a condition of modern lifestyle and diet. Yes, there is a clear genetic basis to insulin resistance, and the first thing we look for in diagnosing it is the presence of diabetes and associated conditions in families. But one look at the modern lifestyle reveals a pattern that explains why this genetic predisposition turns into a pattern of illness.

First of all, we are a sedentary culture. Despite the well-documented relationship between regular exercise and freedom from a variety of conditions from depression to osteoporosis to heart disease, most people do not even manage the 30 minutes of exercise three times per week that is recommended by the American Heart Association. As is described in Chapter 9, exercise plays an important role in lowering blood sugar and insulin levels, thus leading to weight loss and a shift in metabolism away from insulin resistance.

The second issue is our diet. A stroll through any convenience store or supermarket, even the "health food" supermarkets, reveals aisle after aisle of carbohydrate products. Many of these carbohydrate products, like cereals, fast foods, and breads, are advertised as "low fat." While this may be true, the carbohydrates that come from grains are called "high glycemic index" carbohydrates because they tend to stimulate insulin levels. Therefore, the standard American diet (nicknamed "SAD" by some of my nutritionally oriented colleagues) will actually worsen insulin resistance, leading to syndrome X.

By all accounts, people with syndrome X are responsible for a disproportionate number of heart attacks, strokes, circulatory problems, and premature death. This is because of the hardening of the arteries that occurs with increased cholesterol and triglyceride levels in the blood. If physicians are to reverse the high incidence of these serious problems, they will have to pay more attention to syndrome X and its importance in the degenerative diseases of our times.

Glenn S. Rothfeld, M.D.
Regional Medical Director, American WholeHealth
Assistant Clinical Professor, Tufts University
School of Medicine

1

Defining Syndrome X

In all likelihood, you are reading this book because you or someone you know has been diagnosed as having the syndrome of insulin resistance, also called syndrome X. You have concerns and worries, naturally, and probably some fears as well. It can be frightening to walk into the doctor's office with what seem like minor health concerns and walk out with terms like *insulin resistance*, *diabetes*, and *syndrome X* spinning through your mind. Though you might feel singled out right now, you are far from alone. Researchers estimate as many as two in ten American adults have some degree of insulin resistance, the core feature of syndrome X. Without appropriate intervention and treatment, they can develop further health problems.

You do not have to be one of them. Yes, you now have a serious health concern. We do not want to gloss over this reality. But you also have a real opportunity to take control of your lifestyle and your health in ways that can improve both. That you have picked up this book shows you want to make these improvements. You have a lot of questions. While no one has all the answers, this book offers the most current information about this newly identified and potentially deadly health disorder, syndrome X.

This chapter presents an overview of syndrome X—the insulin resistance syndrome—and its various health consequences. Subsequent chapters discuss key aspects of this syndrome in further detail.

What is syndrome X?

In medical terms, a syndrome is a group of health conditions or risks for conditions that, when they occur together, define a particular medical condition. Doctors sometimes describe a syndrome as being like a constellation. When one condition exists by itself, it is like a single star in the sky. When multiple conditions exist together, however, they form an identifiable pattern. In the night sky you might see a pattern of stars as the constellation Orion or the Big Dipper. In your medical records, a pattern of conditions shows a syndrome. Often, syndromes have a key condition at their core.

Syndrome X is a constellation of health conditions that includes type 2 diabetes, hypertension, dyslipidemia, obesity, and risk for early coronary artery disease. In women, syndrome X also includes polycystic ovarian disease, or PCOS. It is likely that further research will reveal additional conditions included in this syndrome.

THE SYMPTOMS AND CONDITIONS OF SYNDROME X

Type 2 Diabetes

Diabetes is a medical disorder affecting the body's ability to metabolize carbohydrates, protein, and fat. There are two major forms of diabetes, so it is important to be clear that only type 2 diabetes is linked to syndrome X. Type 2 diabetes is sometimes called adult-onset diabetes, adult diabetes mellitus, or non–insulin-dependent diabetes mellitus (NIDDM). Type 2 diabetes results from a combination of the body not producing enough insulin and not being able to properly use the insulin it does produce, so that high blood sugar and other metabolic abnormalities develop.

Type 2 diabetes most often develops in adults over age 40,

though it can occur at any age (even in children). It tends to develop slowly. There are typically few signs that type 2 diabetes is developing, though these are the most common:

- increased thirst and urination
- fluctuating changes in vision
- unexplained weight loss
- fatigue
- wounds that don't heal

Many people can successfully manage their type 2 diabetes through diet and exercise. Others take oral medications to help their bodies produce more insulin or make better use of the insulin they produce, and some must take insulin injections.

Dyslipidemia

This hundred-dollar word simply means "abnormal fats." These are the fats that are in your blood, in the forms of triglycerides, phospholipids, and cholesterol. People with dyslipidemia typically have dangerously high levels of these fatty substances, known collectively as lipids. Lipids coat the insides of the arteries, including those that supply the heart itself, with fatty deposits. This narrows the opening through which blood flows. Laboratory tests can measure the amounts of lipids in the blood. Doctors often prescribe a combination of diet, exercise, and medication to try to bring the levels down.

Hypertension

More commonly known as high blood pressure, hypertension causes the walls of the arteries to thicken and stiffen. Hypertension usually has no outward symptoms. The only way to diagnose hypertension is by taking blood pressure readings.

Early Coronary Artery Disease

Every thirty-five seconds, someone in the United States dies from heart disease. That adds up to nearly a million deaths each year. Heart disease claims more lives every year than all forms of cancer and the next six causes of death combined. Once thought of as an age-related problem, heart disease is now recognized as a health concern that can begin as early as the twenties.

Doctors have known for many years that people with diabetes are far more likely to develop heart disease, especially coronary artery disease, at an earlier age than people who do not have diabetes. Only recently have they understood the connection to insulin resistance. Because of this connection, people who have syndrome X often have more advanced heart disease than would be expected for their age.

Coronary artery disease is often a consequence of untreated diabetes, dyslipidemia, and hypertension. As fatty deposits narrow the openings through the arteries, the body responds by raising blood pressure to push enough blood through. Blood clots form on the fatty deposits, narrowing the openings further. This deadly process continues until eventually the arteries are so clogged that fragments of the deposits and blood clots rupture and may break away. Blood pressure continues to rise. The result is a heart attack or stroke.

In many cases, it is possible to halt and even reverse the process of early heart disease development. In fact, many doctors believe as much as 90% of all heart disease, whether associated with syndrome X or not, can be prevented. Lifestyle issues are a key component to succeeding in preventing or reversing heart disease.

Obesity

Many health experts consider obesity the leading health challenge facing America, estimating that 20% to 25% of the population are obese (more than 30% over healthy weight) and 55% are overweight. More than 80% t̶o̶ those who have type 2 diabetes are overweight, and obesity is a key feature of other syndrome X conditions such as hypertension, dyslipidemia, and PCOS.

Researchers are not entirely certain whether insulin resistance leads to obesity or obesity leads to insulin resistance. One theory is that years of lifestyle habits such as overeating and lack of exercise generate changes in the cell functions within the body that cause insulin resistance to develop. An alternate theory speculates that insulin resistance exists as a result of genetic or environmental factors, and obesity is the result of, in part, increased insulin levels in the body. In either case, weight loss improves insulin resistance.

While fast-food eating habits have taken the brunt of the blame for the current weight of Americans, current research suggests an equally likely culprit is lack of exercise. A number of studies show that exercise plus diet is far more effective in reducing both weight and insulin resistance than is dieting alone. So the best course is a combination of nutritional eating and regular exercise, which we discuss in further detail in chapters 8 and 9.

Polycystic Ovarian Syndrome (PCOS)

A leading cause of infertility in women, polycystic ovarian syndrome, or PCOS, affects as many as 20% of women in America. Doctors have known for some time that women with PCOS seem prone to other medical conditions such as early heart disease and obesity but weren't sure of the connection until recent research made the link to syndrome X. About half of those who have PCOS also have other features of syndrome X, most commonly obesity, insulin resistance or type 2 diabetes, and dyslipidemia. Older women who have had PCOS for much of their adult lives are especially prone to early and more severe heart disease.

In PCOS, an imbalance in the normal male and female hormones that can have an effect on menstruation (primarily estrogen, progesterone, and testosterone) causes the ovaries to develop multiple cysts. This can prevent ovulation and cause other symptoms such as hirsutism (excessive body hair). Diagnosis is generally a clinical one that your doctor makes after taking a health history and doing a physical exam. Your doctor will also likely perform blood tests to assess hormone levels and may order an ultrasound examination of the ovaries. Treatment may include medications to regulate hormone levels and, in rare cases, surgery on the ovaries to remove the cysts. Whether or not a woman wants to become pregnant will influence the treatment choices available to her.

How are all of these conditions connected to one another?

While at first glance the constellation of syndrome X may at first seem a collection of conditions that have little in common, research has revealed an unexpected common thread in all of these conditions: insulin—or, more precisely, insulin resistance.

Researchers now know that insulin does not just aid in metabolism but has multiple roles in cell activity. In particular, insulin appears to have a significant role in how both muscle and fat cells function—and specifically, how they use glucose for energy. Resistance to this important action of insulin often causes the body to produce more insulin. This disruption in insulin function and production appears to accelerate certain medical problems such as type 2 diabetes and heart disease.

What causes syndrome X?

As much as we would like to give a simple, straightforward answer to this question, the answer is complex and elusive. No one knows for sure what causes syndrome X. Much of the current research focuses on the insulin resistance connection and on trying to understand what causes insulin resistance to develop in some individuals but not in others. Indicators point to the involvement of both genetic and lifestyle factors.

GENETIC FACTORS

Researchers have discovered a number of genetic mutations in various stages of the insulin cycle that might provide additional information about how and why insulin resistance and related conditions develop. That the features of syndrome X are more common in people with a family history of them also suggests a genetic connection. Research in this area is very exciting because doctors could discover a method that allows them to "turn off" syndrome X before it does any damage.

LIFESTYLE FACTORS

Lifestyle factors seem to be the most significant aspect of syndrome X, particularly inactivity and obesity. While there is evidence that genetic factors predispose certain individuals to obesity, other evidence points to eating and exercise habits. Supporting this are studies showing that people who lose weight, increase their physical activity, and eat nutritiously can reduce their insulin resistance, which in turn lowers their risk for the conditions associated with syndrome X. While many people groan when hearing this, take heart. Here at least is preventive care you can do yourself!

How is syndrome X diagnosed?

Your doctor may suspect syndrome X when your health conditions begin to fall into a pattern for the syndrome. There is no single test that says unequivocally you do or do not have syndrome X. People with insulin resistance have high fasting insulin levels (the amount of insulin in their circulation after fasting for eight to 12 hours is greater than in people who do not have insulin resistance), though "normal" ranges are not well established for general (nonresearch) use. It is not usually necessary to run such tests, which are expensive and often difficult to interpret, to diagnose syndrome X. Most doctors assume that you are insulin resistant if you have a key condition of syndrome X, such as obesity, and will counsel you to be alert for other conditions. If you have more than one condition, such as obesity along with hypertension or dyslipidemia, your doctor may give you the syndrome X diagnosis.

Are some people more likely than others to get syndrome X?

If you are overweight and inactive, you are more likely than someone who is not to develop syndrome X. You are also more likely to develop syndrome X if you are over age 40. Many researchers believe insulin resistance is, to some extent, a normal part of the aging process. In some people it never becomes a problem, while in others it may cause a wide range of medical conditions that extend even beyond syndrome X as we define it today.

People who are obese or have type 2 diabetes, or whose families show a predisposition to these conditions, seem to be at greater risk for developing syndrome X. Certain ethnic populations may also have a higher risk. Native Americans, for example, have the highest incidence of type 2 diabetes in the world. African Americans face an increased risk for hypertension and other forms of heart disease. It's not clear how many of these risks are genetic. Most researchers feel that even when genetics plays a role, environmental factors such as lifestyle habits negatively affect your risk. So even with a genetic predisposition, your risk remains at least to some degree within your control. The best advice is to do what you can to reduce your risks. If you fall into a high-risk group, be especially diligent. Get regular blood pressure checks and blood tests for diabetes.

How do I know if I'm at risk for developing syndrome X?

If you fit any of the categories discussed in the previous section, you are at risk for developing syndrome X. Eventually that covers just about everyone, since risk increases with age. Instead of concentrating on your risk, focus on doing what you can to reduce it. If you are overweight, exercise more and eat less. If you already have one of the syndrome X conditions, take good care of yourself. There is a good chance you can prevent syndrome X from developing if you start your lifestyle improvement plan now.

Is there any way to prevent syndrome X?

Because researchers do not know precisely what causes syndrome X, it is hard to say whether it can be prevented 100% of the time. In many cases, however, the symptoms of syndrome X are directly related to lifestyle factors such as obesity. Cigarette smoking may also play a role, since it is a significant risk factor for developing early heart disease. Many of the factors that we consider to make up "lifestyle" are intertwined. People who eat poorly and exercise little are often overweight, which puts them at risk for the health conditions of syndrome X. Even for those who have a strong family history of these health problems, lifestyle choices can delay the onset of symptoms and help keep them mild when they do show up.

Stay active! This does more to help your body stay healthy than anything else you can do. Muscles that get regular exercise stay well toned. This improves their sensitivity to insulin, which helps them use nutrients more efficiently and effectively. If you stay active, you are likely to eat less as well as to choose more nutritious foods. This helps you maintain an optimum weight. You will have more energy and feel better about yourself. Make regular exercise a part of your daily routine—take a brisk walk around your neighborhood before dinner, go hiking or bicycling on the weekends, join a fitness or sports club. The opportunities are endless. Just keep moving!

My doctor says I have insulin resistance. Is this the same as syndrome X?

Syndrome X is sometimes called insulin resistance syndrome, which is really a more accurate description since insulin resistance is at the core of the syndrome. However, not everyone who has insulin resistance has syndrome X, just as not everyone who has insulin resistance has type 2 diabetes (see Chapter 3 for more discussion of diabetes). If your doctor tells you you are insulin-resistant, however, you are at increased risk for type 2 diabetes and syndrome X. So it is important for you to clarify what your doctor is telling you.

Ask your doctor to explain his or her use of the term *insulin resistance.* You could have test results or other clinical indications that your body is insensitive to the actions of insulin. If this is the case, you most certainly should know about it. If you are overweight, your doctor might suspect insulin resistance as a consequence even without any laboratory tests to corroborate his or her concerns. As later chapters will discuss, there are many ways for you to take control of your lifestyle to improve your health and reduce the effects of symptoms such as insulin resistance.

If I have one of the conditions known to be part of syndrome X, do I have syndrome X?

It is possible, and often common, to have one condition without the others. When this is the case, you do not have syndrome X. To have syndrome X, you must have more than one of the conditions that make up the syndrome.

However, you may be at risk for developing the other conditions of syndrome X if you have only one of them. You could also have other conditions and not know it. Some are difficult to detect until you experience a health crisis. You may not learn that you have type 2 diabetes, for example, until vision changes send you to the eye doctor, who then refers you to your family doctor to test for diabetes. Hypertension (high blood pressure) is another condition common in syndrome X that typically shows no signs of its presence. The potential that such dangers may lurk beneath the surface is why routine health examinations are so important. A typical visit to the doctor nearly always includes a routine blood-pressure check, for example, which helps detect and treat hypertension before it causes a stroke.

If I have one of the conditions known to be part of syndrome X, will I get the others?

Right now, researchers cannot say with certainty that having one condition of syndrome X will lead to developing others. Remember, you must have more than one condition to have syndrome X. It appears that some conditions are more significant when it comes to predicting whether syndrome X will develop. For example, it is common to have coronary artery disease and none of the other conditions of syndrome X. You are at no increased risk for developing syndrome X conditions just because you have coronary artery disease. However, if you have insulin resistance or type 2 diabetes and hypertension or dyslipidemia, your risk of developing early coronary artery disease is much higher. And of course, if you have both type 2 diabetes *and* early coronary artery disease, you do have syndrome X.

With the focus on insulin resistance as the underlying feature in all of the conditions common to syndrome X, finding one condition in the syndrome X constellation should lead your doctor to look for others. This would be particularly important if the one condition you have is insulin resistance or type 2 diabetes. Do you have a family history of diabetes, high blood pressure, or coronary artery disease? These conditions tend to occur more often when there are others in the family who have them too. Are you overweight or over age 40? Syndrome X is most common among people who are both, though being one or the other also increases your risk.

If you have one symptom or condition of syndrome X, you certainly should be aware of the others and discuss with your doctor the possibility that you may have another.

Are there treatments for syndrome X?

Most medical treatment approaches target the individual conditions, combined with diligent monitoring for new conditions. Because obesity is nearly always a common factor, most treatment recommendations include changes in diet and exercise to lose weight. Other conditions, such as hypertension and dyslipidemia, might also require medication.

Some people are interested in natural alternatives (or supplementation) to conventional medical care. While some natural methods, such as yoga and meditation, are certainly helpful, others, like herbal remedies, may have risks. Chapter 7 discusses natural alternatives in greater detail.

Is there a cure for syndrome X?

This is a tough question. In some ways, we can answer yes. Some people are able to gain control over their conditions through diligent lifestyle management and eliminate the harmful effects. And new therapies look quite promising. But for most people, the answer is no. Syndrome X tends to be a lifelong companion that requires ongoing effort and monitoring. The silver lining is that with diligence on your part to minimize adverse lifestyle factors, and regular medical checkups from your doctor, your life can still be long and enjoyable.

2

Center Stage: Insulin's Leading Role

Insulin is a discovery of the twentieth century. Though doctors had suspected a relationship between the pancreas and diabetes for quite some time, they didn't know what the link was. Researchers who were studying the pancreas in the early 1900s identified two types of cells, one of which appeared to produce a substance that affected the amount of sugar in the blood. These cells were called the islets of Langerhans (after the German doctor who first detected them under a microscope) because they were clumped together like little islands scattered among the other cells. Researchers named the substance these cells produced *insulin*, from the Latin word for "island."

In 1921, a young Canadian surgeon, Frederick Banting, and his laboratory assistant, Charles Best, proved the vital function of insulin. They removed the pancreas from a dog and prepared a solution from its dried, ground tissue. When the dog showed classic signs of diabetes, they injected the solution into the dog. The dog made a nearly immediate recovery and stayed alive until the solution made from its pancreas ran out. It was a very exciting discovery for doctors, because until this time a person diagnosed with insulin-dependent diabetes was doomed to die.

Of course, there have been many refinements since Banting and Best's first insulin solution rescued a dog from the

depths of diabetic coma. Most insulin used to treat diabetes
today is genetically engineered ("grown" in a laboratory)
using yeast or bacteria to look and act just like human
insulin. All insulin for treating diabetes is processed under
carefully controlled conditions to assure purity and consistency.

By the 1980s, doctors and researchers were beginning to
notice connections between insulin, type 2 diabetes, and
medical conditions other than diabetes. These other medical
conditions occurred together with such frequency that doctors eventually recognized a syndrome—the insulin resistance syndrome, or syndrome X. Advances in medical
technology spurred new research, which has revealed just
how important insulin is to nearly every function of the
human body. This new understanding of the complex role
insulin plays is leading to new approaches in preventing and
treating insulin resistance and related medical conditions.

What is insulin?

Insulin is a chemical substance called a hormone. Its main
function is to regulate the amount of glucose present in the
body. Though this does not sound very glamorous, it is the
basis for much of cell activity. A gland called the pancreas
makes insulin. The level of insulin in your bloodstream
varies throughout the day. When the body is working normally, insulin levels are highest just after eating and lowest
just before a meal. Insulin serves as a chemical messenger to
cells, telling them to take in more glucose from your blood.
It also instructs the liver to release glycogen (a stored form
of glucose) when blood glucose levels drop. This keeps glucose levels fairly constant, balancing the extremes that occur
with meals on one end of the spectrum and during sleep on
the other end of the spectrum.

Some people who have diabetes take insulin injections up
to several times a day to replace the insulin their bodies are
no longer producing. Since insulin needs vary, people taking

insulin injections must monitor their blood sugar levels to be sure they are taking the right amount of insulin. The amount of insulin in the bloodstream diminishes rapidly as the cells use it to import glucose. It is possible for someone whose diabetes requires insulin injections to receive too much insulin, in which case the blood sugar level can drop dangerously low. The goal with insulin therapy is to maintain as even a balance as possible, avoiding sharp peaks and valleys in both insulin and blood sugar levels.

Recent research has suggested that some foods cause blood-sugar levels to shoot up very rapidly, followed by a corresponding sharp increase in insulin levels. Nutritionists call these foods "high glycemic-index foods." They include potatoes and white rice, as well as items made with refined sugars and grains such as breads and cereals. Some researchers believe this cycle of extremes becomes a contributing factor, over time, to insulin resistance by repeatedly stressing the body's insulin-glucose balance. This balance affects nearly all organ systems. But this area of research is very controversial. Foods with a "low glycemic index," such as fruits and dairy products, may not initiate this cycle of extremes. (For more about the glycemic levels of foods, see Chapter 9.)

What is glucose?

Glucose is the form sugar takes in your body when it enters your bloodstream after digestion. In chemical terms, glucose is a *monosaccharide*, or "simple sugar." It is the fuel source for your cells. Cells can do three things with glucose: They can "burn" it to produce the energy they need to function; convert it into another form of sugar, called glycogen; or use it to make lipids and triglycerides (fatty substances).

It is easy to measure glucose, or blood-sugar, levels. For a precise measurement, your doctor will have you go to a lab to have a blood sample taken. People can measure their blood sugar levels at home by placing a drop of blood into a

machine called a glucose meter. Blood sugar levels provide
an indirect assessment of the amount of insulin in the bloodstream and the degree of insulin resistance that might be present. High blood sugar means there is not enough insulin,
although the absolute level may actually be high. This combination—high blood sugar and inadequate insulin levels—
can have serious physiological consequences, particularly if
untreated.

What is glycogen?

Glycogen is glucose packaged for storage. Your body
stores glycogen in the liver and in muscle tissue. Your body
cannot use glycogen in this storage form. When the amount
of glucose in your bloodstream is not enough to meet the
energy needs of your cells, your pancreas releases another
hormone called glucagon, which the liver uses to convert
glycogen back to glucose.

What is glucagon?

Glucagon is a hormone produced by the pancreas. The
liver uses it to convert glycogen back into glucose to give
fuel to your cells. In this way, glucagon serves to counteract
the effects of insulin. When the blood sugar drops too low
(hypoglycemia), a person can become unconscious. This situation is a medical emergency. Doctors often inject a form
of glucagon to bring the blood sugar level quickly back to
normal.

What is the pancreas?

Looking somewhat like an elongated blob of jelly, the
pancreas weighs about half a pound and stretches along the
back of the stomach in the upper left part of the abdomen.
The pancreas has two distinct functions: It produces the
enzymes your body needs to digest food, and it produces
hormones. These functions are independent of one another.
The pancreas has several key parts.

- **Islets of Langerhans**. So named because they resemble islands and the scientist who first saw them under a microscope was named Langerhans, these clusters are endocrine cells. They secrete hormones directly into the bloodstream. Scientists have identified three kinds of cells in the islets of Langerhans: alpha cells, beta cells, and delta cells.

- **Alpha cells**. These cells within the islets of Langerhans produce glucagon. Diabetes does not appear to affect their functioning directly.

- **Beta cells**. These cells within the islets of Langerhans produce insulin. In type 1 diabetes, the body's immune system begins to perceive the beta cells as foreign substances. It attacks and destroys them, ending the ability of the pancreas to produce insulin. Researchers don't know for sure why this happens, and the destroyed cells do not regenerate. In type 2 diabetes, the beta cells become slow to respond to the body's signals for increased insulin and may also fail to produce enough insulin to meet the body's needs.

- **Delta cells**. These cells within the islets of Langerhans are clearly different from alpha and beta cells, though scientists do not entirely understand their role in health and disease. They produce a hormone called somatostatin, which has many widespread functions in the body.

- **Exocrine cells**. These are the cells that make up the bulk of pancreatic tissue. They are like the field of cells within which the islets of Langerhans cluster. The pancreas's exocrine cells produce digestive enzymes that a network of ducts collects and channels to the pancreatic duct.

- **Pancreatic duct**. This larger conduit is the passageway from the pancreas to the digestive system. It transports pancreatic enzymes to the bile duct, where they mix with enzymes produced by the gallbladder and flow into the stomach.

DIGESTIVE FUNCTIONS OF THE PANCREAS

The enzymes that the pancreas produces are essential for digestion. Most of these enzymes must interact with enzymes the gallbladder produces. This interaction takes place when the enzyme mixture enters the upper portion of the stomach (the duodenum) and encounters stomach acids. These enzymes, along with the acids in the stomach, act on the food you eat to break it down into small chemical substances your body can then metabolize. The pancreas also produces bicarbonate, which flows with the enzymes into the stomach. Bicarbonate neutralizes stomach acid, helping the stomach to settle down and return to normal after its role in digestion is finished.

The digestive functions of the pancreas are generally very stable and continue unimpeded even in the presence of insulin resistance and diabetes. Medical conditions that affect the entire pancreas, such as infection and inflammation, can also affect digestive enzyme production. If this happens, doctors use enzyme supplements until pancreas function returns to normal. In conditions such as pancreatic cancer, in which treatment involves removing the pancreas, this supplementation is necessary for the rest of the patient's life.

HORMONE FUNCTIONS OF THE PANCREAS

Under normal circumstances, insulin and glucagon work in tandem within the body to keep an even level of glucose in the bloodstream throughout the day and night. When one goes up, the other goes down. The body needs this balance and consistent fuel supply to function effectively and efficiently.

A number of factors can affect the hormone functions of the pancreas. One is aging. With increasing age, the pancreas becomes less efficient at producing insulin. Blood sugar levels get higher before triggering the pancreas to release insulin. In addition, cells elsewhere in the body become more resistant to the effects of insulin. Instead of responding with the first signal when insulin "knocks" at the cell wall, the cell may not open itself to take in more glucose until more insulin comes to beat on the door. By that time, blood sugar levels can be quite high. Even after the cells begin admitting more glucose, they are a bit sluggish in burning it to produce energy. The insulin-glucagon balance becomes disrupted, which begins to disrupt other body functions. Age-related changes in the insulin-glucagon balance may explain why people over age fifty are more likely to develop type 2 diabetes than are younger people.

Another influence on insulin production is obesity. Extra fat tissue in the body seems to slow both insulin production and action. This is most likely to happen when a person carries excess weight around the abdomen in the so-called apple body shape. Doctors call this visceral or abdominal obesity, and have known for quite some time that there is a relationship between abdominal obesity and early heart disease. Researchers are not sure exactly what the connection is but believe there is a genetic factor at work because the pattern of obesity seems to run in families. Individuals who have excess abdominal fat but are otherwise not necessarily overweight seem to have a higher risk for both insulin resistance and early heart disease.

People who carry excess weight through the hips and thighs (the "pear" body shape) do not seem to have such an increased risk of early heart disease, though obesity of any kind seems to increase the likelihood of developing insulin resistance and type 2 diabetes. Obesity generally results from unhealthy eating habits (a diet high in calories, simple carbohydrates, and fats) and lack of exercise. This is true even among people with an apparent hereditary connection. Aside from their contributions to weight control, good nutrition and adequate exercise are both necessary for optimal cell function. A balanced diet gives the body the nutrients it needs to generate that fuel, and regular exercise causes the cells to burn that fuel more efficiently. A diet high in simple carbohydrates and fats may give the body too much sugar, some researchers believe, diverting its energy to converting the excess to glycogen.

It is rather like trying to maintain a campfire with only wood chips. The chips will burn, but you will have to keep feeding the fire to keep it going. The fire is in a constant state of burning down or flaring up. A few logs (a mix of soft woods for rapid ignition and hard woods to keep the fire burning a long time) produce a consistent fire that puts out an even level of energy. Careful feeding of this fire with the right mix of logs can keep the fire burning indefinitely. And so it goes with the "fires" of cellular metabolism. Good nutrition provides the balance of fuels the cells need to produce a constant level of energy.

Another factor that influences insulin production and sensitivity is pregnancy. Pregnancy has a tremendous effect on all body systems, and pancreatic functions are no exception. Between 2% and 5% of pregnant women develop a form of diabetes during pregnancy called gestational diabetes, which may or may not go away after pregnancy. Gestational diabetes tends to show up toward the end of the second trimester. Most obstetricians now routinely screen for this condition around the twenty-sixth week of pregnancy. Researchers believe hormonal changes and the increased demands the developing fetus places on the woman's body share responsibility. While some women can control gestational diabetes through diet and exercise, many require treatment with insulin injections.

Between 50% and 75% of the women who get gestational

diabetes will eventually develop type 2 diabetes, compared to about 20% of the general population. Researchers aren't quite sure why this is the case, and do not yet know whether the children of women who had gestational diabetes have an increased risk of developing diabetes (type 1 or type 2). Some studies suggest an infant's weight at birth has an affect on insulin resistance later in life.

Lastly, lifestyle factors such as chronic alcohol abuse and cigarette smoking can affect pancreatic function. Both smoking and alcohol abuse regularly expose body tissues to a multitude of toxic substances. Although cells can fend off permanent damage for a while, eventually their resistance wears down. This reduces their ability to function properly, and leads to premature cell death.

Alcohol is a carbohydrate that metabolizes to glucose after consumption. The resulting spike in blood glucose levels activates the beta cells, which respond by churning out more insulin. Chronic alcohol abuse is also often associated with nutritional deficiencies, which can become severe over time, as well as with abdominal obesity. Alcohol also affects digestive tissue, increasing the pancreas's vulnerability on this front as well. Pancreatic cells can respond to this onslaught by becoming irritated and inflamed, which prevents them from functioning properly. Researchers do not fully understand what role chronic alcohol abuse and its resulting effects on the pancreas have in the development of diabetes. They do know, however, that alcohol has toxic effects on blood vessels.

The relationship between cigarette smoking and insulin production is less clear. People who have smoked regularly over time typically have higher insulin and glucose levels in their blood. Researchers are not sure whether this represents a direct correlation between smoking and insulin production, or if the link is less direct and perhaps comes through effects cigarette smoking has on other body functions. Cigarette smoking is a known risk factor for heart disease, partly because it increases triglyceride and lipid levels.

Though smokers may not be overweight by conventional measures, they often have higher body fat percentages and more abdominal fat deposits. Other lifestyle factors no doubt play a role as well. Doctors know regular exercise is important for not only weight control but also for lowering lipids and triglyceride levels. Smokers are less likely than nonsmokers to exercise regularly and especially aggressively.

How does insulin affect body functions?

Insulin's key function is to regulate the amount of sugar in the bloodstream, which affects a number of body functions.

- **Insulin and glucose.** When insulin action is lacking, such as in insulin resistance, glucose does not get into the muscles to be used for energy production. This results in the liver overproducing glucose, which it makes from the glycogen it stores.
- **Insulin and metabolism.** Severe, chronic deficiency of insulin action can lead to protein (muscle) breakdown.
- **Insulin and lipids (fats).** When insulin levels are insufficient to trigger the liver and muscle tissues to convert glycogen to glucose, the cells must turn to other sources of energy. They begin breaking down fats into fatty acids and triglycerides. Because the entire cycle is out of whack, however, they do not know when to stop. The waste products of this process, called ketones, begin to accumulate in the blood. Ketones are toxic, and quickly lead to a dangerous and potentially fatal condition called acidosis (also called ketosis or ketoacidosis). High levels of insulin also enhance fatty tissue deposits and can influence weight.
- **Insulin and other hormones.** Insulin affects, and is affected by, a number of other hormones, including

glucagon, cortisol, and sex hormones. Though worth mentioning, these interrelationships are too complex to cover in this book. Chapter 5 discusses the relationship between insulin and female sex hormones in polycystic ovarian syndrome (PCOS).

What can go wrong with the body's insulin production?

It is a testimony to the amazing intricacy of the human body that the delicate insulin-glucose cycle functions without problems in most people for many years. Most insulin problems develop over time. However, when things do go wrong, serious consequences result if the problems go untreated.

Type 1 diabetes is the most dramatic insulin problem. The beta cells are destroyed and the pancreas can no longer produce insulin. Type 1 diabetes can progress from early symptoms such as excessive thirst and rapid weight loss to life-threatening ketoacidosis in just a few weeks as hyperglycemia (high blood sugar) results in accelerated fatty acid breakdown. However, the process of beta cell destruction probably goes on for years before any symptoms develop.

The pancreas can also become inflamed as the result of a viral or bacterial infection. Such inflammation may interfere with hormone production, though this is rare. Pancreas functions usually return to normal when the condition causing the inflammation subsides. A possible, though not certain, result is that long-term damage diminishes the ability of the pancreas to produce insulin if the infection destroys pancreatic tissue. Repeated occurrences of inflammation due to other causes such as chronic alcohol abuse can also permanently damage the pancreas, although the beta cells are most often not affected. Such damage affects the pancreas's digestive functions more often than the hormone functions. When this happens, treatment includes supplementation for digestive enzymes and, less often, insulin.

In insulin resistance, the cells in various tissues of the body, particularly in muscles, fat, and the liver, lose their sensitivity to insulin. The pancreas steps up insulin production to compensate, trying to maintain control of blood glucose. If the resistance worsens or the pancreas's beta cells become "tired," the supply of insulin, while still higher than normal, is not enough to maintain normal glucose control. Impaired glucose tolerance, and then type 2 diabetes, when the beta cells are finally "exhausted," result from this situation. Insulin production eventually diminishes altogether (usually over years) and the diabetes becomes more severe. For this reason, longstanding type 2 diabetes often requires insulin treatment as well.

What is insulin resistance?

Insulin resistance defines a sluggish response by cells of the body to insulin's actions. This resistance, or decreased sensitivity, is the key characteristic of insulin resistance and of type 2 diabetes. Insulin normally acts by fitting into a receptor located within the cell, like a key fits into a lock. Once a passage into the cell opens, chemical reactions occur that allow insulin to bring glucose into the cell. The cell uses the glucose to produce energy. This process happens with thousands of cells simultaneously.

In insulin resistance, that part of the receptor-chemical reaction sequence doesn't happen quite right. The insulin "key" doesn't quite fit the cell's "lock" (receptor), and it takes some manipulation for the insulin to get the cell's attention. In an effort to activate the reaction sequence, the pancreas cranks up its production to bombard the receptors with insulin—sort of like beating on the door—when the cell fails to recognize that the "key" is not working. When the insulin finally gains access to pass glucose into the cell, it is as though it has to crawl through an unlocked window instead of entering through the door. Some of the right actions take place, but not all. Cells take in glucose, but the efficiency of actions is altered. Doctors call this situation of "cranked up" (high) insulin levels hyperinsulinemia. Persistent high insulin levels may also cause the number of receptors to decrease somewhat, which is called down regulation, so there may actually be fewer receptors to accept the insulin as well. Hyperinsulinemia develops as a result of insulin resistance and remains as an integral aspect.

Insulin resistance can exist as a medical condition independent of the insulin resistance syndrome, or syndrome X. This is the case when no other features of the syndrome are present.

How does insulin resistance differ from diabetes?

In insulin resistance, especially early on, blood sugar levels may well be normal. Insulin levels are not, however, and because they are not, the entire insulin-glucose balance is out of kilter. Some people who have insulin resistance never develop diabetes, but many do. Because it appears that early intervention through diet and exercise can delay or prevent this evolution, early recognition is especially important.

What is glucose intolerance?

Glucose intolerance is often the stage before diabetes, when the blood sugar is higher than normal but not frankly diabetic. A fasting glucose (the blood level eight to 12 hours after eating) of 110 to 125, or a level between 140 and 199 during an oral glucose tolerance test, means you have glucose intolerance. Insulin resistance accompanies glucose intolerance and type 2 diabetes. Most doctors assume insulin resistance is present when glucose intolerance shows up. In such a situation, an individual is on the brink of type 2 diabetes. Again, lifestyle interventions can keep the condition from progressing, and even return blood sugar levels to normal.

Why is too much glucose a problem?

Too much glucose is a problem for your body in both the short term and the long term. In the short term, excess glucose in the bloodstream can cause fatigue, weight loss, thirst, hunger, skin and vaginal infections, and frequent uri-

nation. High blood glucose levels are toxic for brain tissue,
and can cause unconsciousness and death if not adequately
treated. Such extremes are most likely when insulin deficiency (type 1 diabetes) is the problem. With untreated
insulin resistance and type 2 diabetes, symptoms and consequences are often less severe. A person developing type 2
diabetes, for example, might notice fluctuating vision problems or a general feeling of fatigue.

Longer-term problems include cataracts, blindness, kidney failure, and need for amputations because of serious
lower extremity infections. As glucose leaks into cells and
tissues where it does not belong, it alters those cell and tissue functions. In the eye, for example, high glucose levels
alter the chemical composition of the eye's fluids, creating
distortions in vision. In the cornea, high glucose levels cause
rapid cell growth that produces cataracts. In the body's
blood vessels in the eyes, kidney, and nerves, high glucose
levels distort the function of those blood vessels and the
organs involved, leading to the severe, chronic diabetic complications involving these organs.

As mentioned earlier in this chapter, cells also convert
glucose to lipids and triglycerides. Your body needs these
fatty substances for a variety of purposes—but a little bit
goes a long way. If lipids are excessive, it doesn't take long
for your body's needs to be met. Then your body has to find
someplace to put the excess lipids; there's not much storage
room in the cells that are making them. Because there really
is no designated place for excess lipids; however, your body
gets creative, just like you do when you have extra odds and
ends to stash but no more closet space. You begin looking
for spare space anywhere—under the bed, behind the couch,
and in a pinch, even along the walls in a utility room or
garage. Similarly, your body puts excess lipids wherever it
can find space. It starts dropping lipid cells along the walls
of your arteries and veins. At first, this is no problem. Even
though they are made of fat, lipid cells are pretty thin. When
the lipid layer is just a row or two of cells, it's not in the way.

But when it grows to many rows, it narrows the opening through which your blood is trying to flow and your body's haphazard storage system becomes a health problem.

How are insulin problems diagnosed?

Diagnosing insulin problems is a process of identifying symptoms and abnormal blood test results.

In the case of insulin deficiency or type 1 diabetes, the first hint of a problem usually comes in the form of some common symptoms of high blood sugar—excessive thirst, frequent urination, hunger, weight loss, and blurred vision. Rarely, a person has none of these symptoms but is diagnosed with diabetes when high blood-sugar levels show up on a routine lab test.

With impaired glucose tolerance or type 2 diabetes (high insulin levels), the diagnosis may be less clear at first. A person may have milder manifestations of the similar symptoms. Blood tests can then confirm a doctor's suspicions. It is far more likely for type 2 diabetes to be detected through a routine blood sugar measurement, however, because symptoms are not always obvious or even present.

Insulin resistance syndrome, or syndrome X, is often suspected in a person who has signs of some or all of the features of the syndrome. It is a diagnosis of assumption, based on those features and their association together.

How are insulin problems treated?

Treatment depends on the problem. In situations of insulin deficiency—when the pancreas does not make enough insulin or stops making insulin entirely—doctors prescribe self-administered insulin injections. People with type 1 diabetes always require insulin injections because their bodies have stopped producing insulin. Some people with type 2 diabetes also need insulin injections, though many can control their insulin and glucose levels through a combination of diet and oral (by mouth) medications. Some of these drugs work by stimulating the pancreas to produce more insulin. Others make the cells more sensitive to insulin, which reduces the amount of insulin the pancreas has to produce.

Diet plays a key role in treating these problems and is the primary focus of treatment in type 2 diabetes, impaired glucose tolerance, and insulin resistance. It is important not only to keep insulin and glucose levels within the normal ranges, but also to keep them from widely fluctuating. It is especially important to keep carbohydrate intake consistent, because carbohydrates quickly become glucose in the body.

Doctors also look for any lifestyle factors that could be contributing to a problem with insulin resistance. Many people with insulin resistance and type 2 diabetes are overweight. This is often the result of eating habits and inactivity. Treatment recommendations generally include some kind of regular physical exercise, such as walking and mild to moderate aerobic activities. In addition to helping with weight loss, regular physical activity shapes up cell performance. Cells become more sensitive to insulin, which makes them respond more quickly to insulin that is present in the bloodstream. As a result, the pancreas can back off on insulin production. The key word here is *regular*, however. Intermittent or occasional bursts of physical activity do not have the same effect.

For most people, problems with insulin production or action require lifelong attention. Chapter 3 contains more extensive information about treatment approaches for such problems, including diabetes and insulin resistance.

What happens if problems with insulin production or action go untreated?

Left untreated, such problems tend to get worse. In untreated or undiagnosed type 1 diabetes, of course, the symptoms are usually obvious, and if not treated, can quickly lead to loss of consciousness and death. Untreated type 2 diabetes is unfortunately common because it can exist for years without showing clear signs of its presence. If not treated, or if inadequately treated, type 2 diabetes can result in serious tissue damage to many body systems. Complications can include blindness, extremity amputations, kidney failure, impotence, heart disease, and even death. Untreated or inadequately treated insulin resistance can contribute to these conditions, and often develops into type 2 diabetes.

Doctors can transplant many other organs to cure serious diseases. Why not the pancreas?

Doctors can transplant the pancreas. But an organ transplant is typically done to save a life, performed only when all other treatments have failed. This is a rare situation in the case of insulin resistance and diabetes, which often respond well to less drastic treatment such as medication, diet and exercise, and insulin injections. Organ transplants involve major surgery, and have significant lifetime consequences. As well, organs for transplant are in short supply. A pancreas transplant is most likely to be considered as an option in someone whose pancreas has to be surgically removed because of injury or disease, or in type 1 diabetes when more routine measures have failed. Sometimes a pancreas transplant will be performed when a kidney transplant is required. Organ transplant is not generally an option as a treatment for cancer.

Medical technology may eventually offer other less drastic alternatives that would provide a similar "permanent" fix, however. Gene therapy, in which doctors replace damaged cell material with healthy genetically engineered cells, may be promising. Researchers are also experimenting with "seeding" the liver with healthy beta cells. Such treatments could, if the theory behind them is solid, eventually make transplant or even long-term drug therapy (oral medications or insulin injections) unnecessary.

Despite the potential of such high-tech possibilities, however, the most effective treatment for most problems related to insulin action remains prevention. Except for type 1 diabetes, lifestyle factors play a significant role in insulin-related health conditions (though lifestyle plays an important role in helping those with type 1 diabetes to stay as healthy as possible and to delay complications). Changing these factors—diet, exercise, smoking, drinking alcohol—can delay, reduce the seriousness of, and even prevent insulin resistance. This is true even if insulin resistance and type 2 diabetes seem to run in your family.

3

Metabolic Imbalance: Diabetes

Diabetes is a major health concern in the United States. It is the sixth leading cause of death, and affects an estimated 16 million people. Why "estimated," when there are statistics to pin down the details of nearly every aspect of life these days? Because as many as half of the people who have diabetes do not know it.

THE "HONEY URINE" DISEASE

Before the discovery of insulin in 1921, a diabetes diagnosis was a death sentence. Though even the physicians of ancient Greece and China recognized the symptoms and diseases that result from lack of insulin, they did not know this vital hormone was a key cause. They called it the "honey urine disease" because ants and other insects would swarm to the area where someone with diabetes had urinated. This was one of the earliest diagnostic tests for diabetes. Physicians who observed this then had their students taste a sample of the patient's urine to confirm the sweetness that was the confirming piece of evidence. Medical education, as well as medical knowledge, unfortunately left much to be desired.

Because no one knew what caused this devastating disease, doctors often tried desperate and sometimes cruel treatments to try to save the patient's life. Bloodletting (draining blood from a vein) was also popular, but of course only served to weaken the patient. Even after doctors discovered the blood of a person with diabetes was also sweet, they did not know why or where the sugar came from. Efforts to regulate sugar through diet ranged from forcing patients to eat as much sugar as possible (under the theory that sugar in the blood and urine meant the patient was losing too much sugar) to severely restricting food intake to near-starvation levels (an approach favored by doctors who observed that sugar levels in the blood and urine rose dramatically after eating).

In the 1800s, the condition became known as diabetes mellitus, from the Greek words for "to go through" and "honey sweet." Little else about treatment changed, however, until Canadian researchers Frederick Banting and his laboratory assistant, Charles Best, discovered insulin. The two received a Nobel prize for the work that finally gave hope to people with diabetes.

Then in the 1950s, American physicist Rosalyn Yalow developed a way to detect and measure very small amounts of insulin in the blood. The process, called the radioimmunoassay technique, used radioactive isotopes to measure insulin levels from blood samples. This revealed that while some people with diabetes did not have any insulin at all in their bloodstreams, others did. Some even had apparently normal to high levels of insulin, yet clearly had diabetes on the basis of blood glucose levels. This demonstrated that there were two distinct types of diabetes, and changed the way doctors viewed and treated diabetes. (It also earned Yalow the 1977 Nobel prize in medicine, making her only the second woman in history to do so.)

What is diabetes?

Diabetes is a metabolic disorder involving either the body's production of insulin and/or its sensitivity to insulin's action. The full name for this condition is diabetes mellitus. There are two basic kinds of diabetes: type 1 diabetes, or insulin-dependent diabetes mellitus (IDDM), and type 2 diabetes, or non–insulin-dependent diabetes mellitus (NIDDM). Though the two kinds of diabetes share many common characteristics, they also have distinct differences.

When doctors first realized there were two kinds of diabetes mellitus, they thought the major difference between them was that type 1 diabetes came on suddenly and in childhood, while type 2 diabetes developed slowly and usually in people over age 40. They attributed the presence of insulin in the blood circulation of people with type 2 diabetes to the fact that they were older when they developed diabetes. Reflecting this perception, the two kinds of diabetes were called juvenile onset and adult onset. Research has since demonstrated that while type 1 diabetes occurs primarily in children, adults can acquire it too. The same is true of type 2 diabetes—though it is most common in older adults, children can develop it as well, especially if they are overweight.

TYPE 1 DIABETES: INSULIN-DEPENDENT DIABETES MELLITUS (IDDM)

Type 1 diabetes occurs when the beta cells stop producing enough insulin. Doctors sometimes call this insulin-deficient diabetes, though the more common name is insulin-dependent diabetes. If you look at your medical records, you may find the abbreviation IDDM, which is the old medical term for type 1 diabetes. These terms all mean the same thing—not enough insulin.

Type 1 diabetes often appears to strike suddenly, most often in young people (under age 18). When the disease is clinically manifest, signs and symptoms are usually obvious and grow increasingly more severe. Without prompt medical treatment, which means starting insulin injections, a person with type 1 diabetes could slip into a coma and die. Because the body completely or nearly completely stops producing insulin in type 1 diabetes, insulin replacement is the only treatment at this time, and insulin can only be given by injection or by infusion pump. Doctors believe type 1 is an autoimmune disease, in which, for reasons not quite understood, the body's immune system attacks the beta cells and destroys them.

Though it is type 2 diabetes that is linked with syndrome X, people with type 1 diabetes are at increased risk for developing some of the same conditions, such as heart disease. This is because diabetes, whether the result of insulin deficiency or insulin resistance, has certain effects on body systems that are not related to insulin resistance, but to high blood sugar or hyperglycemia. What distinguishes the connection of syndrome X to type 2 diabetes is the process of insulin resistance, which is not a component of type 1 diabetes. Researchers believe it is high blood sugar levels that, over time, damage blood vessels and nerves. This appears to be a different physiological process than the damage that occurs with insulin resistance.

TYPE 2 DIABETES: NON-INSULIN-DEPENDENT DIABETES MELLITUS (NIDDM)

The primary characteristic of type 2 diabetes is the resistance to the action of insulin. Beta cells continue to produce insulin, though the cells in many of the body's tissues have developed a resistance to its actions. Though type 2 diabetes most often afflicts people over age 40, people of any age can develop it, and it is the most common form of diabetes. In medical terms, type 2 diabetes used to be called non-insulin-dependent diabetes mellitus, abbreviated as NIDDM. Most people with type 2 diabetes can keep their condition under control through lifestyle changes and oral medication, at least in the early years with the disease.

While some people with type 2 diabetes eventually require insulin injections, they are not called insulin-dependent because their bodies do continue producing insulin even if the amount becomes inadequate. Though without insulin injections the diabetes almost certainly will worsen, the person will not move rapidly into life-threatening crisis as will a person with type 1 diabetes who does not take insulin injections. But confusion over usage of the terms "insulin dependent" and "non–insulin dependent" led experts to recommend dropping the use of these terms when referring to the two types of diabetes.

OTHER KINDS OF DIABETES

There are other kinds of diabetes that are quite different from the kinds of diabetes relevant to insulin problems and the insulin resistance syndrome. These other kinds of diabetes are not included in the general perception of diabetes because most have nothing to do with insulin or the pancreas. We will mention them briefly here just to eliminate any confusion.

- **Diabetes insipidus.** Diabetes insipidus has nothing to do with the pancreas, insulin, or glucose. In fact, it has nothing to do with other forms of diabetes at all and is called diabetes only because its main symptoms, excessive thirst and urination, are the same as those for diabetes mellitus. Diabetes insipidus results from a failure of the pituitary gland to produce antidiuretic hormone (ADH). This causes an unquenchable thirst. A person with diabetes insipidus may drink several gallons of water a day and urinate a comparable volume. Treatment includes replacement of ADH.
- **Bronze diabetes.** This very rare metabolic disorder is more correctly known by its medical name,

hemochromatosis. In this inherited condition that affects primarily men, the body deposits high levels of iron in the pancreas, liver, and skin. This gives the skin a bronze hue. The iron deposits in the pancreas can interfere with pancreatic functions, causing diabetes mellitus to develop. Treatment for hemochromatosis is, ironically, the favored therapy of bygone times—bloodletting, known today as venesection. Drawing blood lowers the level of iron in the bloodstream. Secondary treatment may also be necessary for diabetes mellitus, ranging from diet and oral medication to insulin injections.

- **Gestational diabetes.** Gestational diabetes develops in pregnant women who did not have diabetes before pregnancy. There is considerable debate about the causes of gestational diabetes. Most doctors consider it a consequence of the many hormonal changes that take place during pregnancy, and the demands pregnancy puts on a woman's body. Gestational diabetes sometimes goes away after the baby is born. This condition shows up in about 5% of pregnant women, usually around the twenty-sixth week of pregnancy. The most significant hazards of gestational diabetes are to the fetus, which can become excessively large from the abundant supply of sugar and insulin feeding its growth. The baby can also experience low blood sugar after birth as its body struggles to adjust to a much lower level of glucose in its system. Most gestational diabetes responds to diet and exercise. When it does not, the only accepted treatment is insulin injections until delivery, after which the mother's system usually returns to normal. This is considered the safest treatment because oral medications have not been proven safe for the fetus.

What are the signs and symptoms of diabetes?

The two forms of diabetes mellitus have very similar signs (things that are objective and observable) and symptoms (things that are subjective and felt rather than observed). Generally, these are more sudden and severe with type 1 diabetes and may not be present at all with type 2 diabetes.

The common signs and symptoms of diabetes include:

- excessive thirst and drinking
- excessive urination
- unexplained weight loss
- wounds that do not heal
- tiredness and fatigue
- unexplained changes in vision or blurred vision
- excessive hunger
- blood test results showing elevated fasting blood sugar

Clues that diabetes is lurking in the shadows can be harder to detect in type 2 diabetes. More subtle signs and symptoms might include periodontal (gum) disease in a previously healthy mouth, recurrent vaginal yeast infections in women, and dry, itchy skin. Many people only find out that they have type 2 diabetes when a routine lab test turns up a high blood sugar level. Even when the signs and symptoms appear compelling, it takes a blood test to confirm a diagnosis of diabetes.

How is diabetes diagnosed?

The easiest test for diabetes is a fasting blood sugar, for which you go without eating for a period of time (usually overnight) before having your blood drawn. This shows what your blood sugar level is at its lowest point. The normal fasting blood sugar level for an adult is under 110 mg/dL; a result over 125 mg/dL strongly suggests diabetes.

Doctors typically repeat a fasting blood-sugar test to confirm the results of the first test. In combination with other signs and symptoms, this test alone, done on two separate occasions, can be sufficient for a diagnosis of diabetes.

When results are between 110 mg/dL and 125 mg/dL, or other signs and symptoms are vague, your doctor may order a different test called a glucose tolerance test. After you fast overnight, the lab draws a blood sample. Then you drink a sugary mixture and have blood samples taken 30 minutes, 60 minutes, and two hours later. The results show what your glucose level is at its lowest point, how high it rises in response to high sugar intake, and whether your glucose level returns to normal. A result of 200 mg/dL or higher at two hours is a diagnosis of diabetes if confirmed by a second test.

Because type 2 diabetes so often presents fewer or even no clues, many health professionals recommend a screening fasting blood sugar every year after age 45, and earlier if other risk factors such as obesity or family history are present.

What causes diabetes?

Doctors are fairly certain that type 1 diabetes is an autoimmune disorder, even though they do not yet know why it occurs. There is some evidence that a viral infection triggers the autoimmune response, but how and why this happens is not clear. The cause of type 2 diabetes is far more of a mystery, and seems to have more contributing factors. It is not clear whether a single factor is the most important, or whether it takes a grouping of factors to reach "critical mass" that sets the path for type 2 diabetes to develop. Researchers hope to find more answers as they examine the risk factors that seem to make some people more likely to develop type 2 diabetes than others.

GENETIC FACTORS

Researchers continue to explore genetic connections to diabetes. Diabetes does tend to run in families, implying a hereditary link. However, family members tend to have similar lifestyles, too. It can be difficult to separate the two. Advances in medical technology may finally provide researchers with the tools they need to get to the bottom of this issue. Most researchers believe a genetic factor that sets the stage for type 2 diabetes must be present, establishing a predisposition for the condition. Lifestyle factors then trigger this predisposition, allowing type 2 diabetes to develop. Some studies have identified altered genes in the beta cells of people with type 2 diabetes. Other studies are exploring the genetic composition of insulin receptors in the cells of other tissues in the body. The genetic factor seems stronger in type 2 than in type 1 diabetes. However, not all people who have a genetic disposition for diabetes (type 1 or type 2) develop the disease, raising many questions about the role of environment (lifestyle).

THE OBESITY CONNECTION

Most people, probably 85% to 90%, who have type 2 diabetes are obese or overweight. Though this has raised some "chicken or egg" questions among researchers as to whether obesity causes diabetes or diabetes causes obesity, current evidence rests on the side of the former. Supporting this are numerous clinical studies as well as an abundance of practical experience showing that weight loss reduces the signs of type 2 diabetes. Being overweight or obese appears to decrease cell sensitivity to insulin, which reduces the cells' ability to generate energy, which makes a person feel tired. The cycle can progress until it becomes type 2 diabetes, though not all overweight or obese people develop the con-

dition and not everyone who has type 2 diabetes is overweight. And again, doctors do not fully understand the role
genetics plays in the condition's development. It appears
that a person must have a genetic predisposition for type 2
diabetes that is then triggered by lifestyle factors.

In many different ethnic and racial groups obesity corre-
lates very significantly with risk for type 2 diabetes. Those
particularly affected are African Americans, Latinos, and
Native Americans. Researchers are not entirely clear on why
these variations in risk exist. On the other hand, type 1 diabetes is three times more likely to occur in Caucasians than
in any other racial group. There does not appear to be any
correlation between obesity and type 1 diabetes, though
weight management is important after a diagnosis of type 1
diabetes is made.

AGING

Nearly 20% of people over age 65 have diabetes, mostly
type 2. There is compelling evidence that insulin resistance
increases with age. The key challenge for researchers is to
identify the point at which this becomes a problem for the
body. Many body systems change and become less efficient
with age, of course. The risk for a vast number of medical
conditions increases with age, especially among those that
are leading causes of death such as cancer and heart disease.
Again, the issue of lifestyle surfaces. Is insulin resistance an
inevitable aspect of growing older, or an inevitable consequence of less than ideal lifestyle habits? Because diet and
exercise have such a significant effect on insulin resistance,
many doctors believe that healthy lifestyle behaviors can
certainly minimize, if not prevent, insulin resistance with
aging.

What treatments are there for diabetes?

Treatments for diabetes range from lifestyle modifications to insulin injections. People with type 1 diabetes always require insulin injections, while many people with type 2 diabetes can control the condition through diet and exercise. Others with type 2 diabetes use a combination of lifestyle changes and oral medications that normalize blood sugar, some by increasing insulin sensitivity.

LIFESTYLE CHANGES

Regular exercise seems to have a tremendous effect on cell sensitivity to insulin. Even modest activity, such as walking for 30 minutes every day, significantly improves insulin sensitivity. Regular exercise has the added advantage of aiding in weight control. Adding healthy dietary habits to the mix makes even more of a difference. Your body gets the nutrients it needs for optimal functioning, reducing the stress on a number of body systems. Cells can expend their energy for normal functions instead of concentrating so heavily on packaging and storing glycogen and dealing with excess dietary fats.

Some people with type 2 diabetes that is diagnosed early enough can control the condition entirely through diet and exercise. Though this does not cure the diabetes, it decreases the likelihood of complications. Even when medication or insulin is necessary, lifestyle modifications are part of the overall treatment plan. There is much more information about lifestyle habits in Chapters 8 and 9.

ORAL ANTIHYPERGLYCEMICS

Oral antihyperglycemics are drugs taken by mouth that assist the body in reducing the level of glucose in the bloodstream. There are different categories of antihyperglycemics that have different actions. Not everyone responds in the same way to the same drug, so doctors may try several to find what works best. A combination of drugs is most effective in some people.

The last several years have seen an explosion of oral medications for treatment of type 2 diabetes. Although this means there are many more ways to achieve good blood sugar control, it can be confusing. Which diabetes medications are right for whom?

Some medications lower blood sugar by increasing insulin release from the pancreas, including the oldest category of oral medications, the sulfonylureas, and the newest drug, repaglinide (Prandin). The so-called first generation sulfonylureas, introduced in the 1950s, included tolbutamide (Orinase) and chlorpropamide (Diabinese). Because of a lower risk of causing hypoglycemia (low blood sugar), the "second generation" sulfonylureas, glipizide (Glucotrol, Glucotrol XL), glyburide (Micronase, Glynase, DiaBeta), and glimepiride (Amaryl), are more widely used today. With these second-generation sulfonylureas, hypoglycemia occurs more commonly if meals are skipped, in the elderly, or in the presence of kidney or liver disease. Weight gain is another potential side effect. Sulfonylureas are taken once, or at most, twice a day.

Unlike the sulfonylureas, repaglinide, introduced in 1998, is taken before meals and it works when you eat. It is less likely to cause hypoglycemia and weight gain than a sulfonylurea because of the drug's short time of action.

Other medications work by enhancing the body's natural sensitivity to insulin. They help the body's own insulin to control blood sugar better, and are often called "insulin sensitizers." The advantage of these drugs is that hypoglycemia is not a risk, since they do not increase insulin production. Metformin (Glucophage), troglitazone (Rezulin), pioglitazone (Actos), and rosiglitazone (Avandia) are such drugs. Advantages of metformin, a biguanide drug available in the

United States since 1995, include no weight gain (sometimes weight loss), and beneficial effects on blood lipids and other heart disease risk factors. The most common side effects are nausea, indigestion, bloating, and diarrhea, which often improve with continued use or a lower dose. Metformin should not be used in patients who abuse alcohol or have serious kidney or liver disease. It should be used judiciously if congestive heart failure is present. It is taken two to three times per day.

Troglitazone, the first thiazolidinedione drug, was introduced in 1997. The most serious potential side effect of troglitazone is liver inflammation, which may be irreversible. Liver inflammation has not been observed with the other two thiazolidinediones. Research is beginning to discover that this type of drug also may have beneficial effects on blood lipids and other heart disease risk factors. On the down side, thiazolidinediones can sometimes promote weight gain and fluid retention, and increase blood cholesterol. An advantage is once-a-day dosing. Thiazolidinediones can be used in the presence of kidney disease. Researchers have more recently found that the insulin sensitizers may be useful drugs in women with polycystic ovarian syndrome and insulin resistance. (Chapter 5 provides more detailed information about PCOS and insulin resistance.)

Acarbose (Precose), introduced in 1996, and miglitol (Glyset), are in a class called alpha-glucosidase inhibitors. They lower blood sugar by partially blocking carbohydrate absorption from the intestine. Their usefulness is limited by mild efficacy and fairly frequent side effects, including diarrhea, flatulence, and abdominal pain. These drugs are taken with each meal.

The sulfonylureas, metformin, and repaglinide all control blood sugar equally well in most people, and can be used singly, at least for some time. Combinations of medications that work by different means often achieve the best glucose control with the minimum of side effects. Thiazolidine-

diones are most often used in combination with another drug
or insulin, and the alpha-glucosidase inhibitors virtually
always are. Your doctor decides on a treatment after considering not just its effectiveness, but also other possible effects
on weight and blood lipids, the risk of side effects, and cost
and convenience. Oral treatment for diabetes will only be
effective as long as the pancreas is able to produce insulin or
in combination with insulin injections. Talk with your doctor about any questions you may have concerning the benefits and risks of your diabetes treatment.

Don't forget that the cornerstones of treatment for type 2
diabetes are still nutrition and physical activity. *Any* drug
therapy will work more effectively if the diet and exercise
regimen is optimal for weight and glucose control.

INJECTABLE INSULIN

For those with type 1 diabetes, insulin injections are the
only treatment. Some people with type 2 diabetes also need
insulin injections to supplement the insulin their bodies produce. Insulin is injected into the subcutaneous tissue just
under the skin, usually one to four times a day. More injections allow the body to absorb and distribute insulin more
slowly and naturally, reducing the risk of having too much
insulin enter the bloodstream all at once. Insulin can also be
given by a continuous subcutaneous infusion pump which
most closely mimics the natural way that a pancreas works.
Insulin comes in beef, pork, and human variations. Beef and
pork insulin, made from purified cow or pig pancreases, was
once the most common form of insulin but is no longer
available in the United States. This is because the genetically engineered forms are more effective, less expensive to
produce, and have fewer side effects. There are four basic
forms of insulin when categorized according to rapidity of
action.

Very fast-acting insulin, also called lispro (known by the brand name Humalog), takes effect within 15 minutes of being injected and reaches its peak level in about an hour. It lasts for three to four hours. *Fast-acting insulin*, also called regular insulin, begins working within 60 minutes of injection and reaches peak level within two to four hours. It continues to have a diminishing effect for about six to eight hours. Regular and lispro insulins are nearly identical in chemical structure to the insulin that beta cells produce. *Intermediate-acting insulins*, also called NPH or Lente insulins, take about two hours to begin working after injection, and reach peak levels in about six to eight hours. They stay in the system for about 12 to 14 hours and, rarely, as long as 24 hours. *Long-acting insulin,* also called Ultralente insulin, takes four to six hours to start working after being injected, and reaches its peak level around 10 to 14 hours later. Ultralente stays active in the body for about 18 to 20 hours.

Doctors often prescribe a mixture of these forms of insulins to provide the most appropriate coverage for a person's diabetes as well as lifestyle. Because fast-acting insulins act and leave the body so quickly, they are most effective when taken before a meal. Longer-acting insulins maintain a steadier level of insulin in the blood over time but cannot adjust to a sudden increase of glucose such as occurs with a meal. Combining insulins lets most people tailor their treatment to their unique needs and circumstances.

Insulin is measured in units per milliliter. Doctors prescribe insulin, which comes in a concentration of 100 units per millimeter (U-100) for most patients, altering the number of units depending on how much insulin a person needs. Most people who use injectable insulin give themselves injections with a very tiny needle and a syringe made specially for measuring insulin of the 100 units per millimeter concentration.

An increasingly popular method of administering insulin is the injector pen, which uses cartridges preloaded with the proper insulin dose. The injector looks just like a pen, and is easy to carry as well as use. Other injector devices use pressure to "jet" the insulin dose through the skin. Yet another way to deliver injectable insulin is the insulin pump, in which a small plastic catheter placed by a needle stays under the skin. A thin tube connects the needle to a small device the person wears on his or her belt or in a pocket, about the size of a beeper, to send a steady stream of insulin into the body. The pump can also deliver a "shot" of insulin. Though more expensive than other injection methods, the insulin pump offers great convenience for those who use insulin to control their diabetes, and most closely mimics the way a real pancreas works.

How will diabetes change my life?

Diabetes can profoundly change your life. Though this may sound ominous, many people come to regard it as a good thing. No longer a death sentence, a diabetes diagnosis can be the catalyst for a person to alter his or her lifestyle to incorporate healthful eating and exercise habits. What begins as a life-altering event can become a life-affirming experience.

This is not to make light of your situation. Receiving a diagnosis of diabetes can send you reeling, especially if you had few symptoms and learned of your condition incidentally (such as through a routine blood test). Your life has changed, and change always presents challenge. The most important thing for you to do is regain control. Take responsibility for improving your diet and exercising regularly. Take your medication as prescribed. Do all you can to create a healthy environment for your body. Indeed, you cannot go back and undo the past. But you can look ahead to an improved future.

Knowledge and information are essential. Read as much as you can about diabetes and its potential complications. Read about the features of syndrome X, so you know what to watch for and what steps to take to minimize your risk. Talk with your doctor about a comprehensive treatment approach, not just pieces of a treatment plan such as medication. Attend diabetes education classes (and encourage your significant other or family members to go with you). If you are taking medication or insulin, learn as much as you can about how it works and what environmental (lifestyle) factors influence its effectiveness. Identify reliable resources for information about new findings. Your doctor can steer you in the right direction, as can sources such as the American Diabetes Association. And beware the magic bullet—there is no such thing. Do not be fooled by products or services that promise to rid you of diabetes forever. Though there may be a treatment in the future that can do so, it does not exist right now.

How do I monitor my diabetes to be sure my insulin and blood sugar levels stay balanced?

There is no easy way to measure blood insulin levels. The tests to do so are complicated and expensive, and not practical outside a research setting. People with diabetes can and should measure blood sugar levels at home, however, as well as have regular fasting blood sugar and hemoglobin A1c levels (an integrated measure reflecting blood sugar control over two to three months) done at a lab at intervals the doctor recommends. For home use, a small machine called a glucose meter gives a fairly accurate blood sugar reading from a small sample of blood taken from the fingertip. Most people with diabetes check their blood sugar levels one to several times a day. If you are taking medication or insulin, your doctor may instruct you to make changes in your dose based on your blood sugar readings.

In general, people with diabetes should see their doctors at least four times a year just to assess their diabetes. This is in addition to office visits you may have for other reasons. People with diabetes should also receive annual eye examinations from an ophthalmologist (a medical doctor who specializes in conditions affecting vision). Your doctor may have other recommendations or preferences, so this is something you should discuss soon after being diagnosed with diabetes.

Can a woman who has diabetes get pregnant and have a normal pregnancy?

Diabetes can affect a woman's ability to become pregnant, and can also cause complications during pregnancy. Neither of these situations is inevitable, however. There is a strong correlation between insulin resistance/type 2 diabetes and a leading cause of infertility in women, polycystic ovarian syndrome (see Chapter 5 for more information about PCOS). The enormous hormonal changes that take place during pregnancy can affect both type 1 and type 2 diabetes. If you have diabetes and become pregnant, your doctor will monitor your health very closely. If you are taking an oral medication for your diabetes, your doctor should switch you to insulin injections for the duration of your pregnancy.

A potential problem for women who have diabetes when they become pregnant is underweight and overweight babies, both of which increase the risk of a number of health problems in the baby, including stillbirth and birth defects. Appropriate prenatal and obstetrical care can reduce the likelihood of this happening, and greatly improve the odds of a healthy experience for both mother and baby.

Does diabetes affect a man's ability to father children?

Diabetes can affect fertility in men in several ways, and is more likely to do so if the diabetes has been present for a long time. The high blood sugar levels associated with diabetes can damage tiny blood vessels throughout the body. This can affect a man's ability to produce viable sperm. Chronic poor control of diabetes in a man can also result in blood vessel and nerve damage that causes impotence. Once again, prevention is the most effective treatment. Keeping blood sugar levels as constant as possible reduces blood vessel exposure to damaging high amounts of glucose. Sometimes fertility treatments can improve the situation if damage has already occurred, though these can be costly and are not guaranteed to produce results.

What complications can occur with diabetes?

Aside from the constellation of conditions that syndrome X comprises, people who have diabetes are at risk for a number of complications. Many of these can become serious and even life threatening. Yet you can mitigate most by taking good care of yourself. Most complications of diabetes result from chronic exposure to high blood glucose levels. This is one of the most important reasons to minimize wide fluctuations in blood sugar through diet, exercise, and medication or insulin if prescribed.

RENAL (KIDNEY) FAILURE

There are nearly 30,000 new cases of end-stage renal disease, or kidney failure, diagnosed every year. About 40% of them occur in people who have diabetes, making diabetes the largest single cause of this life-threatening disease. About 100,000 people with diabetes undergo dialysis or kidney transplant each year as well. The high glucose levels that occur in diabetes are very damaging to the delicate blood vessels in the kidneys. When enough blood vessels are destroyed, the kidney can no longer function. Kidney failure develops slowly over time, without many symptoms at least at first. Treatment is dialysis (using a machine to filter toxins from the blood) or kidney transplant.

In people who have had type 1 diabetes for five years, or at the time of diagnosis in type 2 diabetes, doctors should order routine lab tests to detect protein in the urine. This is an early sign that the kidneys are not functioning properly. If a urine test reveals protein, medications called ACE inhibitors (commonly used to treat high blood pressure and some forms of heart disease) may delay the progress of kidney disease. Kidney transplant surgery has a high success rate in people who are otherwise fairly healthy, often allow-ing a full return to normal life.

NEUROPATHY (NERVE DAMAGE)

Over time, high blood sugar levels can cause nerve dam-age, especially in the feet. Early symptoms may include an intermittent "pins and needles" tingling sensation, pain, and sensitivity to touch. Doctors believe damage to the blood vessels that supply the nerves is responsible for this neu-ropathy. There is also recent research suggesting that high blood glucose levels interfere with nerve cell metabolism, though this is not conclusive. Impotence is another common form of neuropathy that can affect men who have diabetes.

There are two main categories of diabetes-related neu-ropathy, diffuse and focal. Diffuse is the most common. When it affects the extremities (feet, legs, hands, arms) it is called diffuse peripheral neuropathy. When it affects internal organs and systems (heart, urinary system, sex organs, sweat glands, digestive system) it is called diffuse autonomic or visceral neuropathy. Focal neuropathy affects just certain nerves, such as those around the eyes and face, in the abdomen, or in the pelvis and lower back.

Diffuse peripheral neuropathy that affects the feet can have serious consequences that lead to amputation. When nerve damage reaches the point where sensation diminishes, otherwise minor cuts such as a nick from toenail clippers can become festering and even gangrenous wounds. Because there is no pain, such a wound can become quite advanced before the person notices, especially if it is on the side or bottom of the foot. Good foot care is essential, including careful washing and drying, daily inspections for minor injuries, and comfortable shoes to reduce the likeli-hood of blisters, bunions, and pressure ulcers.

The most effective treatment is prevention by tightly reg-ulating blood sugar levels. A number of studies have shown that keeping blood sugar levels constant significantly reduces the risk of neuropathy and related problems. Early intervention when there is a problem is also essential. A sore spot on the bottom of the foot can ulcerate to the bone in just a few weeks. It sometimes helps to have someone else look at the bottom of the feet carefully every day to check for possible problems. If there is an injury, watch it carefully for any signs of infection (such as swelling or redness), and see a doctor promptly if there are any. Over-the-counter pain relievers often help with discomfort.

RETINOPATHY AND OTHER EYE PROBLEMS

Diabetes is the leading cause of blindness in adults between the ages of 20 and 74. About 20,000 people with diabetes lose their sight each year. Most vision problems are the result of diabetic retinopathy, a condition in which chronic high blood sugar damages the blood vessels in the retina. The retina is the light-sensitive tissue that lines the back of the eye. It collects images and translates them into electrical impulses that then travel along the optic nerve to the brain. When the retina is damaged or destroyed, the eye has no way to send signals to the brain.

Regular eye exams can help detect diabetic retinopathy before it causes blindness. Because retinopathy has few symptoms short of blindness, early detection is critical. Some people notice intermittent blurred vision, which may be caused by blood leaking from damaged blood vessels onto the retina's most sensitive area, the macula. This is called macular edema. Blurred vision can also be caused by temporary fluctuations in the pressure of the fluid in the lens of the eye, so seeing an eye doctor is important to distinguish this transient cause from more severe causes such as retinopathy. As retinopathy progresses, high blood sugar levels feed new blood vessels that begin to grow on the retina. These vessels are very fragile, however, and they rupture easily. Blood leaking from them can cause the appearance of black spots and diminished vision. Left untreated, this bleeding will destroy the retina completely and blindness is the result.

Treatment can involve laser surgery to seal off the leaking blood vessels. If the bleeding has been extensive, conventional eye surgery called a vitrectomy might be necessary. This surgery involves making an incision to remove the blood-clouded fluid inside the eye called the vitreous fluid and replacing it with a saline solution. Neither treatment prevents retinopathy from developing again. Early treatment produces the best results. Waiting too long to seek treatment can result in permanently impaired vision and blindness.

The vision problems that may occur at the onset of type 2 diabetes, often before diabetes is diagnosed, are usually temporary. Your vision gradually returns to what is normal for you as your blood sugar levels and cell metabolism processes normalize, though this can take a month or two. If your vision problems continue after your doctor feels your condition has stabilized, you should have a thorough eye examination by an ophthalmologist.

Is it possible to have diabetes and otherwise be healthy?

Yes, you can have diabetes and otherwise be healthy—if the diabetes is diagnosed early and you manage it aggressively by eating right, remaining physically active, and controlling your blood sugar and any other medical conditions you may have. Get regular checkups to make sure your efforts are having the intended results, and to catch any complications before they cause problems.

How does having diabetes affect other medications I might need to take, such as those for high blood pressure or high cholesterol?

Certain medications may be better for use in a person with diabetes than others. Some drugs aggravate the risks of diabetes, which you want to avoid. In some cases, certain medications may provide added benefits. Any time a doctor prescribes a medication for you, be sure he or she knows you have diabetes and knows what medications, if any, you take for it as well as for any other medical conditions.

Certain types of blood pressure medications, for instance, can potentially aggravate blood sugar control, such as some diuretics and drugs called beta blockers. Medicines called glucocorticoids (such as Prednisone) are sometimes needed to treat asthma, allergic reactions, or some types of inflammation. These drugs typically cause blood sugar to increase. However, if your doctor feels that the benefit of such a drug outweighs the potential risks, something which he or she would weigh very carefully in such a situation, then your doctor may prescribe it. If you really need to take a drug that may interfere with your diabetes management, you will need to watch that aspect of your management more closely.

How does cigarette smoking affect diabetes?

At the risk of sounding like a lecture, we have to say there are no health benefits from cigarette smoking but there are a myriad of health problems. The major concern is that cigarette smoking increases your risk for cardiovascular disease because of its effects on your blood vessels. Diabetes is already a major risk factor for cardiovascular disease, so smoking makes it worse.

How does drinking alcohol affect diabetes?

Drinking alcohol in moderation does not seem to affect diabetes, though it is important to remember that alcohol is a source of empty calories. Alcohol is a carbohydrate in terms of its insulin requirements for metabolism, but is also metabolized as an alcohol. In excess, it can result in either hyperglycemia or, particularly if food intake is inadequate, hypoglycemia.

Chronic alcohol abuse or heavy drinking is another story. It can actually cause diabetes by damaging the pancreas. Chronic alcohol abuse is the leading cause of pancreatic inflammation, which can kill the beta cells that produce insulin. Inadequate nutrition is often associated with chronic alcohol abuse.

Will diabetes go away with weight loss and dietary changes?

If caught early and managed aggressively, the signs of type 2 diabetes can go away. That is, blood sugar can return to and stay at normal levels, and insulin sensitivity can increase. Most doctors believe the condition remains in the shadows, however, and do not consider diabetes to be "cured" even when the signs and symptoms disappear. Because type 1 diabetes is due to a lack of insulin rather than being associated with obesity and insulin resistance, it will not go away with dietary changes. A healthy diet can make it easier to manage, however.

If I have type 2 diabetes, do I also have Syndrome X?

Type 2 diabetes is the core condition that occurs commonly as part of this multimetabolic syndrome. If you have two or more of the other features of the constellation that make up the syndrome as well as insulin resistance or type 2 diabetes, such as hypertension or dyslipidemia, you have syndrome X. If not, you do not have syndrome X, though you are at risk for it.

If I have type 2 diabetes and syndrome X, do I need special treatment?

Many doctors advocate an aggressive prevention effort when you have several features of syndrome X. This is because the various medical conditions appear to develop earlier and become more severe when they exist together. It is important for your treatment plan to target all potential health problems. Fortunately, this is not as difficult as it sounds because many of the same recommendations apply to most of the conditions. Doctors suggest the same diet and exercise changes for diabetes as they do for heart disease, high blood pressure, and high blood lipid levels. A key factor in reducing the risk of complications from any of these conditions is weight loss. Though the different conditions may require different medications, the same lifestyle modifications benefit them all.

4

❧

The Heart Connection

Doctors have known since the 1960s that people with diabetes are more likely to develop early heart disease than those who do not have diabetes, all other factors being equal. Heart disease in people with diabetes is also likely to be more severe. Doctors still do not understand completely why. With type 2 diabetes, one underlying link is insulin resistance.

Heart disease is the leading cause of death in the United States, claiming nearly one million lives a year. In fact, heart disease causes one in two deaths in the United States. More than 58 million people in the United States—20% of the country's population—have heart disease. If you have noticed an emphasis on "United States," give yourself a pat on the back. This is a world record, and not one of which we should be particularly proud. No other country experiences a higher rate of heart disease or deaths from it. The vast majority of heart disease is the direct consequence of lifestyle choices. The typical American diet is high in fat and sugar, while the typical American exercise level is low in activity and frequency. This combination is a catastrophe in the making.

THE HEART AND CIRCULATORY SYSTEM

The heart is an amazing organ. Located behind the ribs just to the left of your sternum, this muscle that gives you life is about the size of your closed fist. It pumps rhythmically and regularly from before your first breath to your last—about two and a half billion times during a typical life. Your heart has four chambers—two that collect incoming blood (the atria), and two that eject outgoing blood (the ventricles). Blood returning from the body goes into the right atrium. When filled, the right atrium releases the blood to the right ventricle, which then pumps it out to the lungs. Oxygenated blood from the lungs returns to the heart's left atrium. When filled, the left atrium releases the blood to the left ventricle, which pumps it out into the body. This tightly coordinated cycle happens 60 to 100 times a minute in a healthy adult.

A vast network of blood vessels—enough to cover 100,000 miles, or four trips around the earth's equator, if all laid out in a straight line—carries the efforts of your heart to every cell in your body—all 300 trillion or so of them. Arteries take oxygen-rich blood away from your heart to the cells and tissues throughout your body. Veins bring the oxygen-depleted blood, bearing carbon dioxide and other metabolic waste, back. Linking the two are the tiniest vessels of all, the capillaries, where the exchange of oxygen for waste takes place. This cycle of renewal happens about 100,000 times a day, and can carry a person through 75 years or more of life.

The force of each heartbeat sends blood through the circulatory system under great pressure to counter the effects of resistance and gravity. The stronger pressure at the start of the heartbeat, when the heart contracts, is the systolic pressure. The weaker pressure at the end of the heartbeat, when the heart relaxes, is the diastolic pressure. Together, these two measurements are your blood pressure. Your blood pressure keeps a steady flow of blood circulating through your body, continually renewing cells and tissues.

The blood that surges through your circulatory system with each beat of your heart contains four elements. Most of your blood volume comes from plasma, a straw-colored fluid that is like the river carrying the other elements. Red blood cells (erythrocytes) contain a substance called hemoglobin, which transports oxygen and other nutrients to your body's cells and picks up carbon dioxide and other metabolic waste to carry away. White blood cells (leukocytes) fight infections. Platelets (thrombocytes) are very sticky and clump together to form clots.

The walls of the arteries are fairly thick and muscular to withstand the high pressures of your heart's systolic beats. This also allows them to contract and relax in synchronization with the pumping of your heart, helping to maintain a consistent blood pressure as well as moving blood through your circulatory system fast enough to meet cell needs for nutrients and waste disposal. A fast flow also keeps the platelets from sticking together and forming clots inside the arteries. These contractions are what you feel as your pulse.

The walls of veins, on the other hand, are thin and flexible. Veins do not contract and relax, though they have strong muscle tone to keep them from stretching too far. Blood flows through veins under much less pressure than it is pumped through arteries. Veins have one-way valves in them to keep blood from flowing back. As blood accumulates between the valves, the pressure forces it to keep moving.

This intricate system works mostly without your awareness. You might occasionally notice a rise in your pulse, such as with vigorous exercise. For the most part, however, your heart and circulatory system quietly work in the background to keep your body alive and well—until there is a problem that demands your attention.

What kinds of heart and blood-vessel diseases are linked to syndrome X?

There are many kinds of heart and blood-vessel diseases. Two in particular are linked to syndrome X: cardiovascular disease and hypertension. Hypertension and dyslipidemia (a disorder of lipid metabolism that can lead to cardiovascular disease) exist as independent medical conditions, and can also contribute to cardiovascular disease. The two forms of cardiovascular disease that are part of the insulin resistance syndrome are coronary artery disease and cerebrovascular disease. Peripheral vascular disease, another form of cardiovascular disease, can develop secondarily as a complication of diabetes or hypertension. These are conditions that damage the arteries and veins. Coronary artery disease involves the blood vessels serving the heart and increases the risk for heart attack. Cerebrovascular disease involves the blood vessels serving the brain and increases the risk for stroke, especially if hypertension (high blood pressure) is present as well. Peripheral vascular disease involves the blood vessels in the extremities, particularly the hands and feet.

What is coronary artery disease?

Coronary artery disease affects the blood vessels that deliver oxygen and nutrients to the heart muscle. Common forms of coronary artery disease include atherosclerosis (thickening of the arterial walls) and arteriosclerosis (stiffening of the arterial walls). In coronary artery disease, cholesterol and other lipids (fats) build up along the inside walls of the arteries. This layer of fatty deposits is called plaque. It narrows the passage through which blood flows, and the blood vessels become stiff. This can slow the flow of blood as well as create bumps and dips, much as rocks do in a river. And like in a river, the blood rushes through some areas and pools in others as it flows over and past the plaque formations.

To further compound the problem, arterial plaque is very sticky. It attracts platelets, which are also sticky and which pile up to form clots. A plaque formation or clot that remains attached to the artery wall is called a thrombosis. When a thrombosis breaks away and enters the bloodstream, it becomes an embolus. And when an embolus reaches the point where it is too large to travel any further in the artery, it creates a blockage called an embolism. A pulmonary embolism can shut down part or all of a lung. A myocardial embolism can cause a heart attack. A cerebral embolism can cause a stroke. These are all very serious, even life-threatening, medical situations.

When healthy, the arteries contract and relax in coordination with the heart's pumping action. When damaged by coronary artery disease, their ability to do this becomes compromised. This results in less oxygen and nutrients being delivered to the heart. As long as nothing strains the heart, it can adjust to its diminished food supply and continue pumping as though nothing is wrong. When a physical or emotional stress signals the heart to pick up the pace, however, the heart cannot respond.

When coronary artery disease affects the heart's ability to function, the result can be cardiac ischemia (impaired cardiac function due to insufficient oxygen to the tissues of the heart) and myocardial infarction (death of heart tissue from lack of oxygen). Ischemia can be present and have no symptoms, or it can cause shortness of breath and a specific type of pain called angina. A thrombosis can also grow large enough to completely block the artery, or break free and lodge in a narrower section of the artery. In either case, the blood stops flowing and heart tissue on the other side of the occlusion (blockage) dies. If enough tissue dies, the heart can no longer function.

In lay terms, a myocardial infarction is a heart attack. It is possible to have a heart attack and experience no or few symptoms, or to feel crushing pain—or anything in between. A heart attack that causes little or no pain is not necessarily less severe than one that causes excruciating pain. All symptoms of possible heart attack—shortness of breath, chest pain or pain that radiates to the left shoulder and arm, nausea, sweating, a feeling of severe indigestion that doesn't go away—require immediate medical attention.

While a good number of other problems can cause similar symptoms, only a doctor can tell the difference.

What causes coronary artery disease?

Many factors contribute to coronary artery disease. One factor is heredity. Coronary artery disease tends to run in families. People whose parents and siblings have coronary artery disease are significantly more likely to develop the condition themselves, even when their lifestyle habits are exemplary. Heredity is considered a fixed risk—it is something you cannot change. If heart disease runs through your family tree, it is especially important for you to eat a healthy diet and exercise regularly. Heredity becomes a risk when members of your immediate family (mother, father, sisters, brothers) have heart disease before age 50. Because the likelihood of developing heart disease increases with age, having family members who died from heart attacks in their eighties and nineties is not considered evidence of a hereditary risk.

Most causes of coronary artery disease are lifestyle matters, however. Fewer than half of all Americans get the minimum amount of regular exercise recommended by health experts—30 minutes of moderate activity, such as walking, four days a week. Even fewer people add the 30 to 60 minutes of vigorous (aerobic) exercise three days a week that heart specialists recommend. And 25% get no physical exercise at all. Regular exercise helps the heart beat stronger and more efficiently, reducing the amount of work it has to do to send blood through the body. It also helps control weight.

Diet is another significant factor in coronary artery disease. The American diet is high in fat. Though doctors recommend that less than 30% of calories come from fat, the typical American diet is 38% fat or more. Unfortunately, there is no way for the body to eliminate excess fat. Your body does not have a way to deal with this excess except to store it. The long, smooth walls of your arteries look pretty inviting for this purpose. Once fatty deposits develop along them you have coronary artery disease.

Not all fat is equal. Fats that remain solid at room temperature, called saturated fats, create more of a problem than fats that are liquid at room temperature, called unsaturated fats. High cholesterol in the diet nearly always corresponds to high cholesterol in the blood. Cholesterol is a lipid, and a primary ingredient of arterial plaque. Though some cholesterol is necessary for cell activities, most American diets contain far more than the body needs. Triglycerides are another form of lipid found both in the diet and in the body.

Too much dietary sugar can contribute to coronary artery disease, too, since the body converts excess sugar into fat. In fact, some health experts now believe dietary sugar is a more significant factor in heart disease than is dietary fat. Chapters 8 and 9 discuss the roles of dietary fat and sugar in greater detail.

What treatments are there for coronary artery disease?

The first line of treatment for coronary artery disease is diet and exercise. Reducing the amounts of fat and sugar in the diet reduces the formation of arterial plaque in the body. Exercise encourages the body to use more energy, which, in combination with lowered dietary fat, can reduce arterial plaque accumulations. Regular exercise also strengthens and tones the muscle tissue of the arteries and veins, making it more difficult for arterial plaque to stick to them.

Doctors may use lipid-lowering drugs to reduce the accumulation of arterial plaque, which in turn reduces the severity of the condition. Other treatments include coronary artery bypass surgery and angioplasty. Coronary artery bypass surgery is open-heart surgery, in which surgeons replace plugged coronary arteries. Angioplasty is a less invasive process in which the surgeon threads a catheter through the body's arteries into the arteries serving the heart. At the end of the catheter is a tiny balloon that, when inflated with a sterile saline solution, compresses the plaque so it no longer blocks the coronary artery. Though these procedures have their risks, they usually succeed at improving the signs and symptoms of coronary artery disease.

How does cigarette smoking affect coronary artery disease?

Cigarette smoking is a prime cause of coronary artery disease. Heart disease is also the leading health consequence of cigarette smoking. Nicotine and other chemicals in cigarette smoke act to stiffen the blood vessel walls and reduce their flexibility. This forces the heart to pump harder and more often to push blood through them. The carbon monoxide in cigarette smoke also blocks oxygen from getting into the bloodstream in the lungs. This means the heart has to work harder to pump more blood to try to meet the body's needs. The longer a person smokes, the more damage is done to the lungs and to the blood vessels. As this damage increases, the strain on the heart grows. This cycle of destruction is particularly devastating when other features of syndrome X, such as hypertension, are present.

I have heard that a drink or two a day is good for your heart. How does alcohol affect coronary artery disease?

In moderation, alcohol consumption probably does not create any further damage. There have been studies that seem to show that drinking one or two alcoholic drinks a day lowers blood cholesterol and has other positive effects on the heart and circulatory system. These studies are not conclusive, however, and have not identified whether the helpful agent is alcohol or another substance. For people who do not have an alcohol abuse problem, an occasional drink seems to be harmless. More than three drinks in a row can directly poison the tissues of your heart as well as other organs, however. And remember, alcohol metabolizes into forms of sugar. These are often excess calories that your body will store as fat. And excess fat is a contributing factor in coronary artery disease.

What is the connection between coronary artery disease and insulin resistance?

From a scientific perspective, the relationship between insulin resistance and coronary artery disease appears strong but is not conclusive. Because there are so many variables that contribute to both coronary artery disease and insulin resistance, it is hard to identify the precise correlation. There is speculation that reduced insulin sensitivity alters cell function to such an extent that all activity is less efficient. This alteration would affect cells throughout the body, since all cells use sugar for fuel and rely on insulin to keep them supplied with just the right level of sugar. When insulin resistance is present, of course, this does not happen. Cells that do not get enough sugar do not produce the energy they need to carry out their functions. This affects a number of metabolic actions, including fat conversion and storage.

Out of the laboratory and in the real world, doctors have long recognized a relationship between insulin resistance and coronary artery disease. They also have observed that the same lifestyle changes benefit both conditions. Though this makes it more difficult for scientists to isolate the causes and relationships of these conditions, it is good news for people who have them.

Can I have syndrome X and not have coronary artery disease?

Yes, it is certainly possible to have the insulin-resistance syndrome and not have coronary artery disease. However, your risk for coronary artery disease is higher, especially if the other features of the syndrome that you have are hypertension or dyslipidemia. Again, the insulin resistance that is at the core of syndrome X increases your risk for coronary artery disease as well.

Can coronary artery disease go away?

It may be possible to reverse very mild coronary artery disease through aggressive changes in diet and exercise. Once coronary artery disease shows symptoms, however, it is not likely to go away entirely.

Many people believe that coronary artery bypass surgery or angioplasty "cures" their coronary artery disease because it eliminates or reduces the plaque accumulations. This is false security. Although indeed you may return from surgery with nearly clean-as-a-whistle coronary arteries, you will be back in the same circumstances within a few years unless you make the lifestyle changes necessary to keep them clean and clear.

What about cerebrovascular disease?

The only difference between coronary artery disease and cerebrovascular disease is the part of the body affected. Coronary artery disease affects the blood vessels serving the heart, while cerebrovascular disease affects the blood vessels serving the brain. Untreated coronary artery disease can cause myocardial ischemia and infarction, while untreated cerebrovascular disease can cause stroke. The mechanisms of disease and the treatments are generally the same for both, with the exception of surgical intervention.

While surgery for coronary artery disease has become almost commonplace as well as highly successful, surgery for cerebrovascular disease is riskier. The blood vessels serving the heart are relatively easy to reach. Even though open-heart surgery requires ribs to be removed and replaced, the damaged arteries are right on the heart's surface. These arteries are big and obvious, and are often easily accessible through angioplasty as well. It is much harder to get to the blood vessels serving and within the brain, even using angioplasty. As well, brain cells begin to die immediately when deprived of oxygen, unlike heart cells, which can survive for several minutes. For these reasons, surgery for cerebrovascular disease becomes a viable option only when other treatment has failed to reduce arterial plaque and blood flow is severely restricted.

What is hypertension?

Hypertension is the medical term for high blood pressure. Blood pressure typically rises and drops throughout the day, fluctuating to some extent with your level of activity. Blood pressure can rise episodically, too, under certain circumstances such as strenuous exercise, anxiety or fear, emotional stress, and cigarette smoking. In these situations, blood pressure usually returns to normal when the event that caused it to rise is over. Blood pressure that stays elevated becomes a medical problem called hypertension.

Hypertension is a serious medical condition. It causes nearly half a million strokes each year and is a major factor in other serious medical conditions such as kidney disease and heart failure. Hypertension is especially dangerous because it seldom shows any symptoms. Treatment that brings the blood pressure back to normal greatly reduces the risk of further medical problems. The damage untreated high blood pressure causes to your body's systems, however, can shorten your life by ten years or more.

Blood pressure readings measure the pressure within your arteries at the point of contraction (systole) and relaxation (diastole) of your heartbeat. Hypertension is defined by blood pressure readings greater than 140/90 in someone without diabetes, and 130/85 in someone who has diabetes. (The first, or top, number is the systolic pressure and the second, or bottom, number is the diastolic pressure.) Because nervousness and stress (physical or emotional) can cause blood pressure to rise, it usually takes several high readings over time to diagnose high blood pressure.

In many people, there is no clear cause for hypertension, though the risk for hypertension increases with obesity and cigarette smoking. People who work in very stressful jobs also may be more likely to get hypertension, though it is not clear what other lifestyle factors, such as diet and exercise, also come into play. And other medical conditions, most notably kidney disease, can cause hypertension. When this is the case, the condition is called secondary hypertension.

How do I know if I have hypertension?

Hypertension usually has no symptoms until it causes a health crisis such as a heart attack or a stroke. Blood pressure is measured with an instrument called a sphygmomanometer. A single blood pressure reading that is high can happen for various reasons. Some people get very anxious when they go to the doctor, which raises blood pressure. This is sometimes called "white coat hypertension." A second blood pressure reading taken after the visit with the doctor may well be within the normal range if anxiety about the visit is to blame for the elevation. If it is not, however, the doctor will usually set up a schedule to have blood pressure readings taken at different times of the day over a period of several weeks. Consistently high readings indicate hypertension.

Blood pressure can go up during pregnancy as well. This is because the mother's body has additional weight and fluid. Health-care providers monitor blood pressure very carefully particularly in the last trimester. Gestational hypertension usually returns to normal following delivery. Treatment focuses on controlling fluid retention as well as physical and emotional stress. A doctor may recommend that a pregnant woman with gestational hypertension limit physical activity and rest with her feet up to help reduce fluid-related swelling and assist the circulatory system in returning blood to the heart.

How is hypertension treated?

Because extra body mass adds to the heart's workload, mild to moderate hypertension often responds well to weight loss. Doctors often recommend lowering salt intake, too. Excess salt draws more fluid from tissues into the bloodstream. This increased volume causes blood pressure to go up.

If weight loss fails to lower blood pressure to the normal range, or if blood pressure readings are above normal levels, your doctor will likely prescribe medication in addition to lifestyle changes. The six common categories of medications that lower blood pressure are called antihypertensives. Most of these drugs are available in various generic and brand-name forms. All brand names mentioned are registered trade names of the companies that manufacture them, and are given as examples, not intended as recommendations or endorsements. There may be many different brand names that are equally effective.

If you are taking medication for high blood pressure, it is very important not to stop taking it suddenly! Doing so can cause your blood pressure to skyrocket, with possibly serious consequences. This is more of a problem with some medications than others, so always check with your doctor if you feel you need to stop taking your medicine.

- **ACE inhibitors.** These drugs are vasodilators— they assist in dilating, or opening, blood vessels. Angiotenin-converting enzyme, or ACE, inhibitors lower blood pressure by preventing the kidneys from making chemicals (angiotensins) that cause capillary constriction. Unlike some other antihypertensives, ACE inhibitors can be used when there are other medical conditions such as diabetes or heart disease. Common brand names include Capoten, Vasotec, Monopril, and Accupril.
- **Angiotensin receptor blockers.** These drugs have much of the same effect as the ACE inhibitors, because they block the receptor through which angiotensin exerts its actions.
- **Alpha blockers.** These drugs are also vasodilators. They block nerve signals telling blood vessels to constrict. Common brand names include Minipress and Cardura.

- **Beta blockers.** These vasodilators are among the most commonly prescribed antihypertensive medications. They are usually effective in lowering moderately elevated blood pressure and have relatively few side effects. Beta blockers affect special cells called beta receptors in the heart itself or in the blood vessels by blocking nerve signals to them. This slows the heart rate and reduces the forcefulness of the heart's pumping action, which lowers the pressure inside the blood vessels. It also keeps the blood vessels more relaxed and dilated, so blood flows through them more easily and with less resistance. Beta blockers are also used to treat other medical conditions such as migraine headaches and angina. Commonly prescribed brand names include Acebutolol, Lopressor, Tenormin, and Inderal.
- **Calcium Channel blockers.** These drugs interfere with the muscle contraction process by disrupting the flow of calcium through muscle cells in the heart and blood vessels. This reduces the effectiveness of the contraction, causing the heart to pump less forcefully and the blood vessels to remain more relaxed. Common brand names include Procardia, Adalat, Calan, Cardizem, and Norvasc.
- **Diuretics.** These are the oldest form of antihypertension medications. Also known as "water pills," diuretics work by increasing the extraction of fluid by the kidneys. This reduces the volume of blood, which in turn lowers the pressure within the blood vessels. A common complaint about diuretics is increased urination. Diuretics can also result in potassium depletion. Doctors often prescribe a mild diuretic drug in combination with another antihypertension drug as a way to attack high blood pressure on two fronts. Commonly prescribed brand names include Dyazide, Maxzide, Bumex, and Lasix.

The choice of medication depends to a great extent on the
individual circumstances of the patient. Many doctors begin
antihypertensive drug therapy with a beta blocker or a
diuretic because these classes of drugs are often successful
with minimal side effects. Different people react to medications in different ways, however, so it is important to inform
your doctor of any unpleasant side effects you might experience. It is also important to have your blood pressure
checked at the frequency your doctor recommends to be sure
that your medication is lowering it as expected. It is not
uncommon to try several medications, or combinations of
medications, before finding what works best for you. Keep
in mind, too, that it takes your body awhile to adjust to a new
medication. Annoying side effects may disappear after a few
weeks.

How do diet and exercise affect hypertension?

A healthy diet and regular exercise generally result in
weight loss, which alone can lower blood pressure. They also
improve insulin sensitivity. In people with mild hypertension,
lifestyle changes can be enough to bring blood pressure to
normal. Even when doctors prescribe antihypertension medications, they recommend diet and exercise to control
weight and provide a healthy environment for your body.

How does cigarette smoking affect hypertension?

Continued exposure to nicotine, one of the main chemicals in tobacco products, makes blood vessels more brittle
and damages their endothelial linings (walls). This can
aggravate hypertension or even cause it over a long period of
time. Cigarette smoking has numerous other adverse effects
on the body as well, which, though they may not directly
cause hypertension, do nothing to improve it. Numerous
studies show that blood pressure typically jumps in a person
who is smoking a cigarette, then returns to normal about 20
minutes after the person finishes. Scientists do not yet know
what role, if any, this cycle of jolts and crashes might have

in hypertension. Long-term effects on vascular stiffness may also be the result of cigarette smoking.

In addition, nicotine is only one of thousands of toxins that enter the body with cigarette smoke, many of which are known carcinogens (cancer-causing agents). No one knows how such exposure affects various organ systems and functions over time. The bottom line is that there are no known health benefits associated with cigarette smoking, and dozens, if not hundreds, of known health complications. If you do not smoke now, do not start (contrary to popular belief, smoking does not help you lose weight—more on this in Chapter 9). And if you do smoke, stop.

How does drinking alcohol affect hypertension?

Alcohol consumption can damage the walls of the blood vessels. This can cause not only hypertension, but also other medical problems such as clot formation.

How does treatment for hypertension change with syndrome X?

The doctor who is treating you for hypertension should know if you have other features of the insulin-resistance syndrome. If your doctor is a family practitioner or internal medicine specialist, he or she is probably also treating you for the other conditions. Some people receive care from a cardiologist (heart specialist) for hypertension and coronary artery disease. Since a cardiologist does not usually treat insulin resistance or diabetes, it is important to coordinate your overall treatment with any other doctors involved in your care. You want each doctor to know all the medications you are taking.

If my blood pressure returns to normal, why do I still need medication?

Once you start taking medication to control your blood pressure, you will probably need to keep taking it for the rest of your life. The key word here is *control*. While antihypertensives bring your blood pressure down, they do not change whatever physiological events have taken place within your body to cause you to have hypertension. Though researchers know a lot about the factors that affect hypertension and have been able to develop drugs to interfere with the mechanisms of hypertension, they do not know exactly what causes hypertension. Future research may reveal more about this. But for the present, medication only controls hypertension, it doesn't cure it.

Can hypertension go away?

Mild hypertension that does not require medication can sometimes go away with the appropriate lifestyle changes. Weight loss is the most effective action. Returning your body to a normal weight dramatically reduces many of the factors that contribute to hypertension. Many doctors are willing to try, and even prefer, a trial period of three to six months to see if you can reduce hypertension through lifestyle changes (diet and exercise) alone. If so, you will need to regularly monitor your blood pressure but may not have any further problems with hypertension. This is not always the case, of course. There are many reasons that hypertension develops, even in people who are physically fit.

If your hypertension requires medication, however, it is less likely to go away.

What is dyslipidemia?

Dyslipidemia is a metabolic disorder in which there are abnormalities in one or more of the blood lipids (fats). There are multiple types of dyslipidemia, grouped according to cause and the particular lipids that are abnormal. Although many have a genetic component, they can be treated at least in part by a healthy, low-fat, low-cholesterol diet and increased physical activity. When this is not enough, effective lipid-lowering drugs are available and can be used.

What causes dyslipidemia?

The causes of dyslipidemia are not quite clear. Poor diet seems to play a significant role, as does poorly controlled diabetes. Because dyslipidemia tends to run in families, researchers suspect there might be a genetic defect that comes into play. In many cases, all three factors coexist.

How is dyslipidemia diagnosed?

The only way to diagnose dyslipidemia is with a lab test called a fasting blood lipid profile. Your doctor may suspect dyslipidemia on the basis of random, nonfasting blood cholesterol and triglycerides levels, but only this more extensive panel of tests can diagnose it for sure.

How is dyslipidemia treated?

In general, treatment for dyslipidemia includes a diet lower in fat and increased physical activity. Depending on the type, treatment may also include lipid-lowering medications that are specific to the type of abnormality.

Drugs called HMG-CoA reductase inhibitors, or statins, are used if the primary problem is elevated total and LDL cholesterol. These drugs may have less effect, but still some, on lowering triglyceride levels. Brand names include Pravachol, Lipitor, and Zocor, among others. Drugs called fibrates, such as Lopid and Tricor, work to primarily lower triglyceride levels. Sometimes the two classes of drugs will be used together to treat both cholesterol and triglyceride problems.

How do diet and exercise affect dyslipidemia?

In many individuals, a healthy diet and regular exercise can correct dyslipidemia, at least in part. This is because your intake of dietary fat influences the levels of lipids (fats) in your blood. Exercise increases cell metabolism, improving the efficiency with which your body can use or otherwise process lipids. A faster metabolism uses more energy, which your body draws in the form of sugar if it is available, and fats if it is not.

How do cigarette smoking and alcohol consumption affect dyslipidemia?

Cigarette smoking and alcohol consumption can affect dyslipidemia in much the same ways they affect cardiovascular disease and hypertension. Cigarette smoking has no positive health benefits, on dyslipidemia or in general. While some studies suggest modest alcohol consumption can reduce the risk for heart-related disorders such as dyslipidemia, much research will need to be done before this is a conclusive correlation.

How does treatment for dyslipidemia change with syndrome X?

If you have other conditions in the insulin-resistance syndrome, especially cardiovascular disease, your doctor may move to more aggressive treatment upon diagnosis. This is because the disease process may be well underway or accelerated. Dietary restrictions on fats and carbohydrates may be more strict, and your doctor may recommend more strenuous regular exercise such as swimming, bicycling, or aerobics, and moderate exercise more frequently for longer periods of time.

If my lipid levels return to normal, can I stop taking medication?

Sometimes it is possible to stop taking lipid-lowering medication once lipid levels return to normal. This is most likely to happen if you have also made significant lifestyle changes to help keep your lipid levels under control without medication. If your doctor tells you that you can stop taking medication, your lipid levels should be closely monitored to make sure they remain normal. It is especially important to continue with a healthy diet and exercise plan.

Does dyslipidemia go away?

If your dyslipidemia is primarily the result of lifestyle factors such as obesity, poor diet, and inactivity, it is possible for it to go away with appropriate treatment. Again, it is essential to continue a healthy diet and exercise regimen to keep your lipid levels normal. Dyslipidemia that is the result of a genetic defect, which is fairly common, is not so likely to go away, but may get somewhat better with a healthy diet and exercise regimen.

If I have hypertension or dyslipidemia, or my doctor says I have syndrome X, does that mean I have heart disease?

Hypertension and dyslipidemia can lead to heart disease in that, if untreated, they will most likely progress to the point where heart damage takes place. Having hypertension or dyslipidemia does not mean this progression is inevitable, however. Early and effective intervention can halt and even reverse whatever minimal damage has already occurred, and continued diligence in lifestyle choices can keep heart disease at bay.

Having hypertension or dyslipidemia does increase your risk for developing heart disease, however. Each risk factor you have—each condition within the syndrome X constellation—compounds your risk exponentially. This means that while having one risk factor, such as hypertension, may increase your risk fourfold, having two (such as hypertension and dyslipidemia) may multiply your risk by ten times or more. And if you already have insulin resistance or diabetes, you have at least one risk factor. Any other condition you develop then significantly increases your risk.

All this being said, do not panic if you have several conditions within the insulin-resistance syndrome! You still have great opportunity, by making smart lifestyle choices and receiving regular health checkups and medical care, to delay and perhaps prevent heart disease from developing. No one's health future is carved in stone. Each and every positive change you make—and maintain—in your life has a positive effect on your health and well-being. The whole point of becoming more knowledgeable about syndrome X and its constellation of conditions is to improve your influence and control over contributing factors. Just as adding a condition exponentially increases your risks of heart disease and other complications, so does decreasing one lessen them. Even if you cannot make all your signs, symptoms, and conditions go away, you can reduce the extent to which they affect your life and your health.

5

～

For Women Only:
Polycystic Ovarian Syndrome (PCOS)

Polycystic ovarian syndrome, or PCOS, can be emotionally devastating for women who have it. They typically experience obesity, acne, infertility, irregular menstrual cycles, and hair growth on the face, chest, and back (hirsutism). PCOS can damage self-esteem as well as cause medical problems. While as many as 20% of women may have cysts in their ovaries, only about 6% to 10% of women actually have PCOS. While ovarian cysts are quite common, they usually do not cause any symptoms or problems. For a diagnosis of PCOS, at least one of the syndrome's clinical signs must also be present. PCOS is sometimes called Stein-Leventhal syndrome, after the two doctors who in 1935 first identified a condition in women marked by hirsutism, obesity, and irregular menses. As doctors learned more about the syndrome and made the connection to polycystic ovaries, they began to refer to it in more clinically descriptive terms.

What is Polycystic Ovarian Syndrome (PCOS)?

PCOS is a metabolic disorder that affects the female reproductive system. The key characteristics include irregular menstruation and male pattern hair growth (hirsutism). *Polycystic* means "many cysts," and the ovaries in women with PCOS are typically large and full of cysts (though often this is only apparent with a pelvic exam or pelvic ultrasound). Many women with PCOS are insulin resistant, and many women with PCOS are also overweight or obese, which increases the insulin resistance. To understand PCOS, it helps first to understand the normal female reproductive system.

THE FEMALE REPRODUCTIVE SYSTEM

The organs of the female reproductive system are located in the lower abdomen. The pear-shaped uterus rests just above the pubic bone. The uterus, sometimes called the womb, becomes home for a developing fetus if pregnancy takes place. This hollow, muscular organ has a remarkable ability to stretch and distend to support a growing fetus. On each side of the uterus, attached by short stems of tissue, are the ovaries. These roughly egg-shaped glands produce the ova, or eggs. Each ovary contains about a million ova at birth, though only a fraction of them will mature to be released during ovulation (about 300 from both ovaries combined). The ova reside in microscopic cavities within the ovary called follicles. When mature, an ovum is about a tenth of a millimeter in size, not quite large enough to be visible to the naked eye. Providing passage for the eggs into the uterus are the two fallopian tubes, which extend from the top of the uterus on each side. Leading from the bottom of the uterus to outside the body is a muscular, flexible channel called the vagina.

The cycle of producing and releasing an ovum is called ovulation. At ovulation, the ovary "shoots" a ripened ovum from its follicle, much as a flower might discharge a burst of pollen. Tentacle-like structures called the fimbriae gently pull the ovum toward the opening of the fallopian tube. If sperm are present in the tube, the ovum becomes fertilized and continues its journey into the uterus, where the developing embryo implants itself into the endometrium, or thickened lining of the uterus wall. If the ovum is not fertilized, it passes into the uterus and out through the vagina with the sloughed-off endometrium during menstruation.

This entire process—ovulation through menstruation—is called the menstrual cycle, and its biological purpose is procreation. It is a woman's cycle of fertility. A normal menstrual cycle represents a complex process of hormonal actions that takes place every 28 to 35 days. The cycle begins when the pituitary gland releases follicle-stimulating hormone, or FSH. FSH does just what its name implies—it stimulates the ovary's follicles to ripen an ovum. Usually several ova mature, though just one is released at ovulation. Ova that mature and are not released are resorbed back into the ovary's tissues. It takes 10 to 14 days for the ova to ripen, during which time the follicles are producing and releasing the hormone estrogen. Estrogen causes the walls of the uterus (endometrium) to thicken and increase their blood supply in anticipation of pregnancy. Another hormone called luteinizing hormone, or LH, signals the follicle to release a mature ovum. The vacated follicle then produces a hormone called progesterone, which prepares the thickened endometrium to receive an embryo for implantation—much as you might add soil neutralizers and fertilizers to your garden just before you plant seeds.

If fertilization occurs, the resulting embryo burrows into the endometrium to begin its 38-week odyssey from cluster of cells to newborn infant. This implantation stimulates the follicle to continue producing progesterone, initiating the intricate hormonal and physiological changes of pregnancy. If fertilization does not occur, there is no implantation and the follicle stops producing progesterone. Estrogen production drops off as well. The endometrium sloughs from the uterus as a bloody discharge, carrying the ovum with it out of the body via the vagina. This bleeding phase is the menstrual period, which typically lasts five to seven days.

Women who have PCOS nearly always have irregular,

and typically infrequent, menstrual cycles. Some may menstruate every six to eight weeks, while others menstruate only once or twice a year. Periods may be extraordinarily heavy and long, or brief and scanty. Cysts and hormonal imbalances often prevent the ovaries from releasing eggs, resulting in "empty" cycles and infertility.

FEMALE AND MALE HORMONES

Though we tend to think of male hormones in terms of men's bodies and female hormones in terms of women's bodies, in reality both men and women have male and female hormones. It is the balance of their presence that produces what we identify as male or female physical characteristics. Women's bodies have predominantly female hormones, and men's bodies have predominantly male hormones.

The primary female hormones are estrogen and progesterone. (There are actually several forms of estrogen, though for simplicity we will refer to them collectively as estrogen.) A woman's body dramatically increases production of these hormones during puberty, which usually takes place between the ages of ten and fourteen. Puberty signals the transition from child to adult, and begins when the pituitary gland starts increasing the production of hormones called gonadatropins that cause the ovaries to increase the secretion of estrogen. This causes numerous physical changes in the body, including breast development, pubic hair growth, and the onset of menstruation. Puberty concludes when all of these secondary sexual characteristics are complete, generally by age sixteen to eighteen. During puberty, it is normal for menstrual cycles to be irregular and anovulatory. An adolescent girl may have a period every six to eight weeks, or every four weeks for a few months and then not again for two months. Her ovaries may or may not release mature ova.

A woman's ovaries also produce tiny amounts of male

hormones, called androgens. The adrenal glands also produce small amounts of androgens. The most important of these is testosterone, which influences bone and muscle development as well as sex drive. Men have much higher levels of testosterone (produced by the testes) in their bodies than women do, which gives men their facial and body hair and larger, stronger bones and muscles. In women, testosterone levels are normally very low. With PCOS, the ovaries and the adrenal glands produce more androgens, most notably testosterone. The ovaries may also produce less estrogen and progesterone (female hormones). The resulting imbalance is responsible for many PCOS features.

What are the signs and symptoms of PCOS?

The signs and symptoms that cause most women with PCOS to seek medical attention include:

- infrequent and irregular periods
- inability to become pregnant (infertility)
- male pattern of facial and body hair (hirsutism)
- acne

Many women with PCOS also have insulin resistance, and some may even have type 2 diabetes. The doctor's examination usually reveals two additional signs of the syndrome: multiple cysts in the ovaries and elevated levels of male hormones in the blood. Occasionally, the cysts cause abdominal discomfort or even pain, though most women do not know they have ovarian cysts until an exam reveals their presence. As well, the symptoms of PCOS are often more severe when the woman who has it is overweight. Doctors believe this reflects the involvement of insulin resistance, which also is often more pronounced in people who are overweight.

It is possible to have one or even two of these symptoms and not have PCOS. However, having two or more of them is cause to suspect the presence of the disorder. Symptoms may vary in severity and tend to worsen without treatment.

What causes PCOS?

Doctors have known of PCOS as a defined medical condition since 1935 (when it was known as Stein-Leventhal syndrome, after the doctors who identified it). Until recently, it was considered a gynecological problem involving an imbalance between male and female hormones in the woman's body. Then doctors began noticing that many women with PCOS also had some degree of insulin resistance. Researchers now believe the underlying cause of most cases of PCOS is a defect, probably genetic, that causes the ovaries to be more sensitive to insulin's effects. When insulin levels are higher than normal, this stimulates the ovaries to produce more androgens (male hormones), even if ovarian sensitivity is normal. This eventually establishes the hormonal imbalance that results in the symptoms of PCOS.

Though research seems to support a genetic connection, environmental factors such as diet and exercise clearly affect the severity of PCOS in many women. Some women see their symptoms completely disappear with weight loss and regular activity, and most see at least some level of improvement in their symptoms. This is further support for the role of insulin resistance, which also improves with lifestyle changes such as weight loss, exercise, and nutritional eating habits. Like the other conditions of syndrome X, PCOS is most likely a blend of genetics and environment.

My gynecologist told me I had an ovarian cyst, but it went away on its own. Does this mean I have PCOS?

Ovarian cysts are quite common, especially in younger women whose menstrual cycles are not yet well established. Having an occasional ovarian cyst is not a sign of PCOS. A cyst is a swelling or growth. Many women have ovarian cysts from time to time and are not even aware of them, because most ovarian cysts are painless and go away within two or three menstrual cycles. Other cysts can be quite painful, and may have to be surgically removed.

Ovarian cysts are actually follicular cysts. Such cysts grow in a follicle, one of hundreds of microscopic cavities in the ovary where eggs develop. A follicular cyst contains fluid and may grow as large as ten centimeters (about four inches). Depending on its location, a large cyst may cause pain during intercourse or with certain movements. More than 95% of follicular cysts are resorbed and disappear. Follicular cysts nearly always develop one at a time.

Cystadenomas are cysts that develop from other tissues in the ovary. These cysts can grow much larger than follicular cysts, though usually do not cause pain until they get quite big. Most are filled with fluid or with a gelatinous substance. Though cystadenomas can disappear on their own, they are more likely to require surgical removal. Dermoid cysts grow from ovarian germ cells (cells that produce eggs) and contain an odd mix of tissue bits including skin, hair, bone, and sometimes teeth. Dermoid cysts are firm and do not go away on their own. Unlike other ovarian cysts, a dermoid cyst often shows up on an X ray. Doctors are likely to suggest surgery for cysts that do not go away within a few months to be sure they are not cancerous.

The cysts that develop in PCOS are different from any of these other ovarian cysts. Most importantly, they occur in numbers. A polycystic ovary can easily have a dozen cysts. Like simple follicular cysts, these develop in the follicles where the ovary produces eggs. Unlike simple follicular cysts, however, the cysts common in PCOS occur in numbers. As many as a dozen may be present at the same time and occur repeatedly. This eventually damages the follicles, interfering with the ovary's ability to produce eggs. This is a contributing factor in the infertility many women with PCOS experience.

How does insulin affect female hormones and ovulation?

There are two kinds of cells in the ovary that produce male and female hormones. Theca cells produce the male hormone testosterone and granulosa cells produce the female hormone progesterone. High levels of insulin, such as those that occur with insulin resistance, stimulate theca cells to secrete more testosterone. This creates an imbalance in the sex hormones that disrupts menstrual cycles and causes increased hair growth in male patterns (such as on the face).

Higher than normal insulin levels also appear to affect the pituitary gland's production of luteinizing hormone (LH). LH influences estrogen and progesterone (the female hormones) production. This further disrupts the cycle of ovulation and menstruation.

The disrupted menstrual cycles are usually anovulatory, which means no ovum is released and the cycle is "empty." Conception cannot take place because there is no ovum to fertilize. This is why infertility is so common in women with PCOS. Some evidence indicates that bringing insulin levels down through weight loss and medication can restore the balance of sex hormones and allow fertile menstrual cycles to take place. Any damage that has occurred to the follicles and the ovaries as the result of repeated multiple cysts may still prevent the release of mature ova, however.

How is PCOS diagnosed?

The doctor arrives at a diagnosis of PCOS by comparing the history of your symptoms and experiences with the findings of a physical exam and lab tests. Because each of the features of PCOS can have other causes, the doctor will evaluate these to rule them out. Disorders of the adrenal and pituitary glands, for example, can cause excessive or unusual hair growth. Typically, the doctor will use blood tests to measure hormone levels, and sometimes an ultrasound examination to confirm the presence of ovarian cysts. An ultrasound is not always necessary to make the diagnosis.

How is PCOS treated?

Many of the symptoms of PCOS respond well to weight loss. Both hirsutism and acne often diminish and may even disappear when PCOS is mild. In some women, normal ovulation also returns. Doctors believe such improvements result from improved insulin sensitivity within the body's cells. This in turn reduces insulin's interference with sex hormone production and actions.

For most women, medical treatment for PCOS is most effective when it combines hormones, insulin-sensitizing medications, and sometimes androgen-blocking drugs, which partially block the effects of androgens on the skin and hair follicles. The particular combination that is most effective for you depends on the severity of your symptoms and how well you tolerate the medications. Some people experience side effects with certain insulin-sensitizing medications but not with others. It can also take time to find the level of hormone therapy that produces the desired results without undesired side effects. It might take some experimentation and time to find the right blend for you.

Some symptoms take longer to go away than others, even with medical treatment. Acne typically clears up within a few weeks, while hirsutism can take six months to a year to even begin to disappear. Cosmetic aids such as electrolysis to remove unwanted hair can help minimize hirsutism until treatment restores the hormonal balances in your body and your body hair patterns return to normal.

HORMONE MEDICATIONS

Birth-control pills are a common form of hormone treatment that provide relief of PCOS signs and symptoms in some women. Birth-control pills that are most effective are low-estrogen formulations. High-progesterone pills can make the hirsutism worse because progesterone can act like an androgen.

Another hormone treatment might involve taking andro-gen-blocking drugs such as spironolactone and cyproterone. Only spironolactone is available in the United States. Flu-tamide is not FDA-approved for this use, but it is sometimes used as an androgen-receptor blocker. Some doctors may prescribe finasteride (Propecia), which also is not FDA-approved for this use. It blocks the enzyme 5-alpha reduc-tase, which converts testosterone into the more active-on-skin form of androgen, dihydrotestosterone, or DHT, so it can sometimes be helpful with hirsutism. Drugs such as clomiphene and gonadatropins are sometimes prescribed for women with PCOS who want to become pregnant. They restore fertility by stimulating ovulation and normal men-strual cycles. These drugs also increase the possibility of multiple pregnancy (two or more babies) by overstimulating the ovaries to release multiple eggs.

The androgen-blocking drugs and the 5-alpha reductase inhibitors should not be used if a woman is trying to get pregnant—they can cause birth defects if the fetus is a male. For this reason they are almost always prescribed with birth-control pills.

INSULIN-SENSITIZING MEDICATIONS

The insulin-sensitizing drugs prescribed for type 2 dia-betes work by enhancing the body's sensitivity to insulin at the cell level. (Chapter 3 discusses these medications in detail.) Those that appear to be most effective in reducing the signs and symptoms of PCOS are metformin (Glu-cophage), troglitazone (Rezulin), pioglitazone (Actos), and rosiglitazone (Avandia). One of the common side effects of the latter three medications can be weight gain. Metformin is not associated with weight gain, so is often a first choice. However, metformin can sometimes cause unpleasant side effects including nausea, indigestion, and diarrhea. These side effects often improve after taking the medication for a few days. Sometimes a lower dose is easier to tolerate. One positive side effect with metformin is that it may reduce blood lipid levels.

Doctors typically use insulin-sensitizing medications in type 2 diabetes to increase the body's ability to appropriately use insulin, with the goal of lowering blood sugar levels. Women who have PCOS may not have type 2 diabetes. Insulin-sensitizing drugs such as those mentioned here do not have any effect on blood sugar levels in people who do not have higher than normal fasting blood sugar levels. (Other medications to treat high blood sugar may lower blood sugar in people whose fasting blood sugar levels are normal, creating a potentially dangerous situation of hypoglycemia. These medications are not used to treat PCOS.)

SURGERY

A surgical procedure called open wedge resection of the ovary, which involves cutting a polycystic section out of the ovary, was once a common treatment for severe PCOS, though it is seldom used now. This kind of surgery has a high risk for obstructions that would block the fallopian tubes, causing infertility. Occasionally a reproductive specialist will recommend laparoscopic surgery to remove particularly large or bothersome cysts as a treatment for infertility. Laparoscopic surgery involves inserting a flexible, lighted tube (a fiberoptic laparoscope) through a small incision. The surgeon manipulates tiny instruments at the end of the tube to remove tissue with minimal damage to surrounding areas. There is usually little or no internal scarring with laparoscopic surgery, significantly reducing the risk of an obstruction developing later.

If PCOS is causing heavy bleeding in a woman who is near menopause, a gynecologist might recommend hysterectomy (surgery to remove the uterus). This is because repeated heavy bleeding can cause severe anemia. Hysterectomy is not an option for younger women who might want to become pregnant, because once the uterus is removed, there is no way to carry a pregnancy.

LIFESTYLE CHANGES

Like the other conditions in the syndrome X constellation, PCOS responds well to healthier eating habits and increased physical activity. Many women with PCOS find it difficult to lose weight, which has caused some doctors to speculate that weight gain is a consequence, as well as a contributing factor, of PCOS. (Chapter 8 discusses the many factors that influence weight control in greater detail.) Many women with PCOS find it easier to lose weight after they begin taking insulin-sensitizing medication, adopt a diet lower in fats and carbohydrates, and add regular exercise to their daily activities.

If I have PCOS, can I become pregnant?
There are many causes of infertility. PCOS is the leading cause of anovulatory infertility—infertility that results from no egg being released during the menstrual cycle. If this is the primary cause of your infertility, than it is possible that correcting the hormonal imbalances present in PCOS could restore your fertility and you could become pregnant. However, infertility is a complex situation. Even if PCOS seems to be the primary cause, there could be other factors involved.

If you have PCOS and you want to become pregnant, you will want to work closely with a specialist in reproductive medicine who has a comprehensive understanding of PCOS and its relationship to insulin resistance. Most reproductive specialists have such an in-depth understanding; however, general practice obstetricians and family practitioners may not. Though PCOS is by no means rare, it is a complex metabolic disorder. While anovulation is the leading cause of infertility in women, not all anovulation results from PCOS. In fact, most anovulation has no identifiable cause. PCOS represents a highly specialized area of medicine, and research studies are steadily producing new knowledge.

There are concerns about the possible effects that the insulin-sensitizing medications now being used to treat PCOS might have on a developing fetus. Doctors do not prescribe these medications for women who have type 2 diabetes and become pregnant. No one knows what effects they could have if they are being taken at the time of conception. This creates a bit of a tightrope as far as treatment goes. The most effective and most uncomplicated way to restore fertility is to restore the body's hormone balance, including insulin. However, this has unknown potential risks. So doctors often prescribe hormone-based drugs commonly used to treat infertility to aid women with PCOS who want to conceive. These drugs, too, have their risks—most notably, overstimulation of the ovary, resulting in multiple pregnancy.

If you have PCOS and you do *not* want to become pregnant, do not rely on your condition to function as birth control, however. The body's hormonal balances are very intricate, and it is possible that you could occasionally ovulate and release a viable egg. If you have intercourse during ovulation that releases a viable ovum, you could conceive even though you may have had years of nonfertile menstrual cycles. Discuss your birth-control preferences and needs with the doctor who is treating your PCOS.

I have heard that taking hormones can cause cancer. Is it safe to take them for PCOS?

Most health experts agree that the benefits of hormonal balance far outweigh the probably very slight increase in risk of certain kinds of cancer that taking medically prescribed hormones may subject you to. In particular, female hormones (estrogen) offer increased protection against heart disease and osteoporosis, two medical conditions that dramatically increase in women past menopause.

Some evidence indicates that continued hormone imbalance increases the risk of certain kinds of cancer as well. Some studies indicate that the abnormally thick and blood-rich endometrium common in untreated PCOS is itself a risk factor for endometrial cancer (cancer of the walls of the uterus). Women with untreated PCOS are also more likely to experience heavy bleeding and other difficulties during menopause. PCOS may be a risk for later development of ovarian cancer.

As with any treatment plan, discuss all of your options with your doctor. Talk about the risks and advantages of the treatment approach your doctor recommends, and try to identify the reasons your doctor makes this recommendation over other treatments that are available. Obtain as much information about your condition and possible treatments from reputable sources so you can make decisions based on knowledge rather than emotion.

Does PCOS go away after menopause?

Yes, PCOS often does go away after menopause because the ovarian follicles stop growing. This will end symptoms such as hirsutism and acne. However, insulin resistance is likely to persist.

It does not concern me that I could be infertile and my symptoms are mild enough that I can live with them. Do I still need treatment?

Because individual circumstances vary, you should discuss your symptoms and treatment options with your doctor. Doctors do not like to prescribe medication when it is of questionable value. If your doctor suggests hormones or insulin-sensitizing medications, there is likely solid clinical evidence that your body needs them for optimal health. The body's hormone balance is quite delicate, and there is still some question that hormones can influence the development of certain types of cancer.

One factor to consider is whether your symptoms will worsen over time if left untreated. This is often the case, particularly when insulin resistance is present. PCOS symptoms seem to progress, sometimes even with treatment. Another consideration is the link between PCOS and other conditions of syndrome X, such as hypertension and dyslipidemia. Women with PCOS are far more likely to develop these conditions as well, with potential health consequences beyond infertility. The most effective way to reduce or prevent these other more serious medical problems is through early intervention and treatment of the less serious conditions. Choosing not to treat PCOS because the symptoms are mild is not much different from deciding not to treat diabetes because the blood sugar levels are not that high. These syndrome X conditions are all progressive. Failing to intervene early is a sure prescription for problems later.

Can insulin resistance or type 2 diabetes cause PCOS and other fertility problems?

Researchers now believe insulin resistance is often at the center of PCOS. The high levels of insulin in the bloodstream that are typical in insulin resistance as well as type 2 diabetes stimulate the ovaries to increase their androgen production. This directly affects fertility by creating an environment within the body that is hormonally hostile. Elevated androgens suppress ovulation. They alter the hormone balance, interfering with the menstrual cycle. PCOS is the single most common cause of infertility due to anovulation. Doctors have found that treatment with insulin-sensitizing drugs alone (without hormone medications) restores fertility in some women, further supporting this connection.

What is the connection between obesity and PCOS?

Most, but not all, women with PCOS are at least overweight, if not obese. Being overweight increases the magni-

tude of the insulin resistance in most cases, elevating the
insulin levels, which, in turn, further stimulate the ovaries.
Though being overweight often is associated in and of itself
with high insulin levels, the entire picture is not totally clear
as to how obesity and PCOS interact. It is almost a vicious
cycle—as you gain more weight, you become more insulin
resistant, and you gain more weight perhaps in part because
of the insulin resistance.

Women who are overweight or obese and who have
PCOS typically have the "apple" body fat–distribution pattern in which they carry most of their excess weight through
their midsections. This is the same pattern typical in other
conditions in which insulin resistance is a factor. However,
it is important to stress that not all women who are overweight have PCOS, whether they are "apples" or "pears."

How is PCOS linked to syndrome X?

Insulin resistance, recently discovered to be present in the
majority of women who have PCOS, provides the first link
to syndrome X. Other links include the tendency of women
with PCOS to also have, or to develop, type 2 diabetes,
hypertension, and dyslipidemia. Even before doctors understood that insulin resistance was a key factor in PCOS, they
knew that women who had the disorder had a much higher
likelihood of developing type 2 diabetes and early heart disease than women who did not have it.

If I have PCOS but don't have type 2 diabetes, do I have syndrome X?

The likelihood is fairly high that a woman who has PCOS
also has other features of syndrome X, even if type 2 diabetes is not one of them. Insulin resistance, dyslipidemia,
and hypertension are common in women who have PCOS.
Women who have PCOS are also at high risk for developing
type 2 diabetes. This risk diminishes when treatment brings
PCOS and insulin sensitivity under control.

If I have PCOS, am I likely to develop syndrome X?

It is likely that you will develop other conditions of syndrome X if you have PCOS. It is likely, in fact, that you already have at least early indications of some of these other conditions if you have been diagnosed with PCOS, because PCOS itself is a constellation of conditions. As with other syndrome X conditions, insulin resistance is a key feature. Some women who have PCOS have normal fasting blood sugar levels, leading to the conclusion that they also have normal insulin levels.

If I am a woman who has syndrome X, do I have PCOS?

You do not necessarily have PCOS if you are a woman with other syndrome X conditions, unless you have the specific symptoms of PCOS such as irregular menstrual cycles and some degree of hirsutism. Nor are you necessarily more likely to develop PCOS as a consequence of having other syndrome X conditions. You are, however, at increased risk for early heart disease as a result of untreated conditions such as dyslipidemia or hypertension.

Will conventional treatment for PCOS reduce my risk of developing syndrome X?

Before doctors recognized the insulin-resistance connection, treatment for PCOS focused on restoring the hormonal balance of the body through hormone supplements. Though this approach sometimes managed the symptoms, it did not address the underlying issue of insulin resistance, so probably had little or no effect on the development of other syndrome X conditions. Such an approach is not as common today as it was five years ago; most specialists now add insulin-sensitizing medications and lifestyle changes to treatment plans for PCOS. Lifestyle changes in areas such as eating habits and exercise unquestionably influence hypertension, dyslipidemia, and diabetes.

Is there special treatment for PCOS when syndrome X is suspected?

It is possible for a woman to have polycystic ovaries (multiple ovarian cysts) and not have PCOS. This would be the case if testing ruled out the other aspects of the disorder, and multiple cysts in the ovaries were the only sign. In this case, medical care would focus on treating the cysts and most likely would not include any effort to influence insulin sensitivity.

When other syndrome X conditions are present, treatment should include some effort to improve insulin sensitivity. Diet and exercise alone might accomplish this, or insulin-sensitizing medications might be necessary. If hypertension or dyslipidemia is also present, it would be necessary to treat those conditions as well.

Will treatment for insulin resistance or type 2 diabetes "cure" PCOS?

Treatment can relieve most or all of the symptoms of PCOS. This does not necessarily mean the disorder is cured, however. PCOS symptoms tend to come back if treatment ends. It is possible for treatment to keep PCOS under control to the extent that symptoms remain at bay. As women age, symptoms of PCOS can sometimes improve.

Does syndrome X have any effect on male hormones in men?

At this time, it does not appear that insulin resistance has any effect on male hormones in men. There is no obvious "male version" of PCOS, though some researchers are exploring a possible connection between insulin resistance and male pattern baldness. There is some evidence that men who have typical male pattern baldness are also likely to have insulin resistance. It will take more research to determine if this connection is coincidental or clinical.

6

~

Living with Syndrome X

Learning that you have some or several features of the insulin-resistance syndrome changes your picture of your health. In fact, it can leave you feeling that your entire life has been turned upside down. You now have a chronic medical condition—a health problem that, though likely to improve with treatment, may be with you for the rest of your life. Because you are no doubt anticipating that will be a long time, this can be (and often is) a startling recognition.

It is not always easy to live with chronic medical conditions. Their presence changes your life and your lifestyle. It is common to feel powerless about this. But you should instead feel empowered, for you actually have a great deal of choice about these changes. You cannot turn back the clock to some magical moment in your life just *before* the stage was set for your diabetes or hypertension or PCOS to develop. There is no such moment. So it serves very little purpose to look back. Your mission now is to look forward.

Your life now has new routines and different characteristics. You might take medication once to several times a day, or even insulin injections. Nothing passes your lips without lighting up a mental scoreboard tallying fats, carbohydrates, and calories. You have aches and pains where you did not remember having muscles. As hard as it may be to accept, this is all good news. You did not lose your life to a heart attack, your body to a stroke, or your vision to untreated diabetes. You found out that you have health problems you can, with modest effort, control.

Doctors often recommend a combination of lifestyle changes and medications in an effort to both relieve symptoms and improve health. This is your treatment plan. Each individual's situation is unique, and your treatment plan takes into consideration numerous factors that make you different from someone else who has the same health problem. It is important to follow your doctor's treatment plan. If there are parts of it that you do not understand or agree with, or find you cannot comply with after trying them for a time, discuss alternatives with your doctor. Do not just stop something because it is unpleasant or takes too much effort.

Other chapters in this book cover in detail the treatments specific to the individual conditions of syndrome X. This chapter examines the collective issues of treatment and the issues of living with chronic health conditions.

What medical care do I need?

Your doctor will tell you how often to have lab tests, blood pressure readings, or office visits. If you do not know or cannot remember, ask. Keep these appointments current. It is important to have regular follow-up care with any chronic condition, particularly if you are taking medication for it. Many prescriptions require a doctor's approval before they can be refilled, which is one way your doctor can keep track of how long you have been taking the medication and when you need follow-up care or tests.

What can I expect from medical treatment?

With appropriate medical treatment, you can expect much of your life to be normal—recognizing, of course, that "normal" now includes healthy eating habits and regular exercise. Medications are very effective in controlling the symptoms of hypertension, dyslipidemia, insulin resistance, and type 2 diabetes. Medication is less reliable in producing results with PCOS, though certainly may result in significant improvements in symptoms.

What you *cannot* expect from medical treatment is a miracle cure. You are likely to have your medical condition and at least the risk for some others, for the rest of your life. Nor can you expect medications alone to carry the load. Lifestyle issues are integral to syndrome X and its conditions. Think of medication as a way to enhance lifestyle changes, not the other way around. You can expect to gain control over your medical conditions with appropriate treatment. With treatment, you also can expect to reduce your risk for developing early heart disease, and for developing other conditions within the syndrome X constellation.

I'm worried about taking all these medications. Don't they have potentially serious side effects?

Many people worry about side effects, which can range from mildly unpleasant to harmful. All medications, whether over-the-counter or prescription, carry the potential for side effects. This has nothing to do with the drug's inherent safety. Medications undergo rigorous testing before the Food and Drug Administration (FDA) approves them for use. FDA standards evaluate how well a drug does what its developers and researchers say it does, and also what happens when a drug does not quite measure up. Stringent manufacturing procedures produce drugs that are of uniform strength.

There is always the possibility that a problem can crop up after a drug has been in use for a while that did not reveal itself during research and trial use. Drug trials use relatively small, though statistically significant, sample populations. Participants are people who have the condition the drug is supposed to help. Some receive the medication being tested, and some receive a placebo (looks just like the real thing but has no active ingredients). Neither knows which they are taking, real or placebo, and usually the doctor or researcher administering the medication does not know either. This is to prevent any unintentional bias from influencing the participant's responses and reactions. Though these trials note every sign and symptom observed and reported, sometimes the trial group is not diverse or large enough, or the study is not long enough, to reveal side effects that are rare or a result of long-term use. When this happens, the drug is pulled from the market or placed under strict prescribing guidelines.

DIFFERENT DRUGS FOR DIFFERENT NEEDS

Despite how much the same all human bodies are, every body is unique. You can see this just by looking at the people around you. Just as no two people look the same on the outside, no two bodies are quite identical on the inside. What works for the person who was sitting next to you in the doctor's waiting room may not work for you, even though it sounds like you have exactly the same health problems. You do not have the same bodies, medical histories, or life circumstances. Indeed, the doctor might make the same recommendations and prescribe the same medications. But this is because he or she feels this is the best course of treatment for you, not because this is what worked for someone else.

SIDE EFFECTS

A side effect is an action a drug has that is not its primary effect. Your doctor or pharmacist should discuss both the benefits and possible side effects of any medication prescribed for you. What does your doctor expect this medication to do for your condition, or how will it help? Most medications have known side effects that occur in certain people or under certain circumstances. Some people who take insulin-sensitizing drugs, for example, experience nausea and intestinal distress. This does not mean the drug is not working as intended. It may mean your body needs a period of time to adjust to the regular intake of this substance, which is usually the case. Or it could mean that your body would better tolerate a different medication that has similar actions.

Side effects can be positive or negative. Many insulin-sensitizing drugs have both positive and negative side effects. Metformin's primary action is to increase the sensitivity of the body's cells to the action of insulin, which it does quite effectively in most people with insulin resistance or type 2 diabetes. Among its positive side effects are the ability to lower some blood lipids and to sometimes result in weight loss. Negative side effects include digestive upset and, rarely, kidney or liver problems. Negative side effects are sometimes called adverse reactions.

Most pharmacies now provide patient information handouts that describe a medication's intended actions, positive side effects, and negative side effects in detail. If you do not receive such material when you get a prescription filled, ask for it. Though this material is a bit technical, it is supposed to be written in language the average person can understand. A pharmacist can answer any questions you have or explain information that you do not understand.

DRUG INTERACTIONS

Drug interactions may be a concern for you if you are taking multiple medications. A drug interaction occurs when two or more medications have different, and often unintended, effects when taken together. This is a particular risk if different doctors prescribe your medications. One way to minimize potential problems is to make a list of all the medications you are taking, and update it every time there is a change. Carry this list with you, and show it to each doctor when you have an appointment. You might also show the list to the pharmacist when you pick up a new medication. Many pharmacies keep computerized records that show what medications you have purchased. If the pharmacy is part of a large chain, these records often show prescriptions filled by any store within the chain. The computer programs that many pharmacies use automatically alert the pharmacist to potential interactions, which the pharmacist and the doctor can then evaluate.

Remember to include any over-the-counter medications or herbal remedies that you are taking as well. These, too, are considered drugs and can interact with each other or with prescription medications. Substances you take regularly are the most likely to cause an interaction. An occasional ibuprofen tablet taken for a headache is not likely to make a difference, for example, though taking ibuprofen four times a day for arthritis certainly could. Other common over-the-counter products include antihistamines (for allergies and cold symptoms) and antacids or products for indigestion. Read the label! The instructions for use often include warnings about possible drug interactions with particular medications. If you are not sure about taking an over-the-counter product with your prescription medications, talk with a pharmacist.

What happens if I choose not to take the medications my doctor prescribes?

Doctors prescribe medications to treat medical conditions because they believe, based on the evidence of your symptoms and knowledge acquired through extensive research, that the benefits far outweigh the risks. If you object to taking medications, discuss your concerns with your doctor. There may well be information available that can set your mind at ease about the treatment plan your doctor recommends.

If your symptoms are mild, you might be able to bring them under control through lifestyle changes. This will require diligence on your part to strictly comply with the dietary and exercise recommendations. Your body is relying entirely on the changes you make, without any assistance from medications. You cannot eat nutritiously and exercise every day for three weeks and then take a week off if you want to control your condition through behavioral and lifestyle changes (just as you cannot take your medication every now and then, and get the same results as if you took it as prescribed).

Making such significant lifestyle changes is by no means an impossible task, of course. Many people are successful in turning their lives around in terms of developing habits that promote health. The challenge is often that you not only must implement positive changes, but that you must also simultaneously eliminate negative habits. Because your behaviors represent a lifetime of practice, you may engage in many of them without conscious thought. This is not just true of eating and exercise habits, but also of any activities you do on a routine basis such as brushing your teeth or driving a car. You do not usually think of each step as you perform it. Making changes in any of these long-term habits, whether driving or eating, requires conscious attention to the steps you have become accustomed to taking automatically. Some people may develop syndrome X conditions even though they do have apparently healthy lifestyle habits. This probably reflects the genetic aspects of these conditions. For these people, lifestyle remains important though is not likely to completely control the conditions and their symptoms.

Just as taking medications has risks, so too does choosing not to take them. Making the choice to forego medication could set you on a course of near-certain complications as your conditions become more advanced and your symptoms more severe. Your choice not to take medication shapes the future of your health just as surely as your choice to take them. Remember, your doctor has prescribed the medication for you because he or she believes it is the best course of treatment. Be sure you have all available information before making your decision. Knowledge truly is power. There are many sources for reliable information. You can find books as

well as articles in health and medical journals at public and
medical or nursing school libraries. Your doctor's office
probably has brochures and information sheets about health
conditions and treatment options. Your pharmacist can provide patient information material about medications. National
organizations that support research and education about specific conditions are also a good resource, especially for
information about the latest research. (There is a list of some
of these in the back of this book.) Unfortunately, some
sources provide unreliable information, particularly on the
Internet. Be especially wary of personal websites that discuss one individual's problems with medications or success
with alternative treatments.

How do treatment approaches for syndrome X differ from treatments for the individual conditions?

In many respects, treatment approaches are the same for
the medical conditions common to syndrome X as they are
for those conditions when they occur independently. Someone with dyslipidemia will most likely receive lipid-lowering medication and instructions for nutritious eating and
regular exercise. Someone with hypertension will receive
antihypertensive medication and similar instructions for
lifestyle modifications. The picture really does not change
much when two or more conditions are present together,
though treatment may be more aggressive if insulin resistance or type 2 diabetes is among them.

Knowing you have multiple features of syndrome X is a
red flag that you are at risk for developing more severe
health problems earlier in life than someone who does not
have these symptoms. Because lifestyle factors are so critical in each syndrome X feature, they take on major significance when multiple features are present. The double
cheeseburger and fries that wants to become your lunch will
gurgle through your digestive system if you eat it. It will
contribute to elevated blood lipid, insulin, and sugar levels—which, as you now know, are responsible for numerous

health problems within the constellation of conditions that form syndrome X.

It is important to treat each component of the insulin-resistance syndrome, and also to be aware of what effects that treatment may have on other components. Some medications work better in combinations than others. Some medications aggravate other conditions, while others have beneficial side effects. Sometimes a particular medication works well for a while, then begins to lose its effectiveness. Regular blood tests and office visits will monitor you for this. Occasionally new medications come onto the market that may be more effective, or have fewer negative side effects.

If treatment brings one of syndrome X's conditions under control, how does that affect the remaining conditions?

In some people, improving insulin sensitivity (reducing insulin resistance) results in general improvements in other syndrome X conditions such as dyslipidemia and PCOS. Any beneficial lifestyle change, such as losing weight, eating healthier, and becoming more physically active is likely to improve the other conditions to some extent. In general, the most effective medical approach is to treat each existing condition of syndrome X and regularly monitor for the development of others. Often there is some overlap in treatment, so one aspect can affect several or all of the conditions you have. Medications that increase insulin sensitivity and lifestyle changes that result in weight loss are good examples; they affect the insulin resistance that underlies syndrome X conditions in most people.

Will treatment make me "good as new"?

Treatment usually reduces, and can sometimes eliminate, symptoms. Medication and weight loss, for example, can bring blood pressure to within normal ranges. Likewise, medication, weight loss, and regular exercise can bring blood glucose levels to normal, too. Doctors do not usually consider this result a "cure" in the sense that you will no longer have to deal with this condition. Some people whose symptoms are mild are able to stop taking medication once their condition stabilizes and stays within normal ranges. The conditions most responsive to treatment are mild forms of hypertension, dyslipidemia, and insulin resistance. If your doctor does give you the go-ahead to stop taking medication, be sure to maintain the lifestyle changes that helped your condition improve.

How do I know if treatment is doing any good?

You should see improvement after a reasonable amount of time with a particular treatment approach. How much time and how much improvement depends on the condition and the severity of your symptoms. As hard as it is, be patient. You did not develop these conditions overnight, and they will not improve or go away overnight. Steady, consistent improvement is the main goal—even if the pace is slow. Remember, the conditions of syndrome X are intricately related. It takes time not only to treat the individual conditions, but also to unravel their connections within your body.

REASONABLE EXPECTATIONS

When you and your doctor discuss your treatment plan, talk about what you should expect. It often takes months to notice improvement with conditions such as dyslipidemia and PCOS, while hypertension may show significant improvement within a few weeks. Some aspects of the conditions retreat faster than others as well. Certain lipid levels may show improvement within just a few weeks with treatment for dyslipidemia, while others may take six months or longer to nudge downward into normal ranges. PCOS is a particularly challenging condition from a treatment perspective, because there are so many variables involved. Ovulation and regular menstrual periods may return within a few months of treatment, while it could take a year or more for body and facial hair to return to normal.

Be sure you understand what your medications can and cannot do for your condition. There is a tendency to expect medications to do all the work in improving symptoms, as antibiotics do when you have an infection. Unlike infections, however, syndrome X conditions all have significant lifestyle factors that contribute to their symptoms. Taking medication without making the necessary changes in your eating and exercise habits is like bailing water from a capsizing boat without plugging the leak.

SIGNS THAT ALL IS NOT WELL

There are clues you can watch for that will tell you not all is well. Your symptoms should begin to improve, at least somewhat, once your treatment has been underway for a month or two. Minor but unpleasant side effects with medications should go away within a few weeks. If this does not seem to be the case, contact your doctor. You might do better with a different medication dose, or a different drug altogether.

Sometimes treating one condition successfully brings other medical problems to the surface. Be sure to let your doctor know if you begin experiencing symptoms you did not have before you started your treatment plan. Sometimes it becomes necessary to adjust medication doses after significant weight loss. This should be among the aspects of your care that your doctor is regularly monitoring. If you lose more than 10% of what you weighed when you started taking medication, ask your doctor whether you should continue at the same dose.

It is important to pay close attention to your vision, especially if you have diabetes. Many people experience vision changes before their diabetes is diagnosed, and most of the time vision returns to normal within a few months of starting treatment. If it does not, or if your vision seems to get worse despite treatment, you should get a thorough eye exam by an ophthalmologist. A key symptom of diabetic retinopathy, which can cause blindness, is sudden dark patches in your field of vision. This is an emergency; it indicates bleeding on your retina. Without immediate medical attention (and usually eye surgery), you are at great risk for losing your vision. Diabetic retinopathy is most likely to occur in someone who has untreated or undertreated type 1 or type 2 diabetes.

What symptoms should I watch for as possible indications that other syndrome X conditions are developing?

Each condition of syndrome X has potentially serious consequences. Though these are usually more of a problem in people who are not receiving treatment, they can happen even with treatment. Your doctor will check for evidence of advancing cardiovascular disease during your regular checkups, as well as any developing complications related to diabetes. Warning signs for you to watch for include:

- **Chest pain.** This is a very late symptom of coronary artery disease, and could signal a heart attack. Closely monitoring blood lipid levels and blood pressure are part of monitoring for the progression of coronary artery disease. Always seek medical attention right away for chest pain.
- **Sudden severe headache, tingling, or numbness on one side of the body.** These can be symptoms of stroke, a potential consequence of hypertension. Prompt medical attention is crucial, and can mean the difference between a few hours in the emergency room and a few months in rehabilitation. There are drugs that can dissolve clots to restore blood flow to the brain, drastically reducing or eliminating any damage.
- **Fluctuating changes in vision, or black spots in your field of vision.** These symptoms can indicate

macular swelling or retinal bleeding, two serious problems that result in blindness unless treated promptly. These symptoms may rarely be the first clue that diabetes is present, especially in someone who has neglected regular medical care.

If you have more than one of the conditions of syndrome X, you are of course at increased risk for developing others. These may not have overt symptoms. Hypertension and dyslipidemia, for example, seldom have noticeable symptoms. Your doctor will regularly check your blood pressure and your blood lipid levels to monitor for these conditions. Your doctor will also regularly check your fasting blood glucose level to monitor insulin resistance.

Is it inevitable that I will develop all of the syndrome X conditions?

Nothing is inevitable. In fact, there is a good chance you can avoid developing further syndrome X conditions through lifestyle changes and appropriate medication.

What can I do to reduce my risk for developing additional syndrome X conditions?

We cannot stress enough the importance of a healthy diet, regular physical activity, and maintaining a normal weight. It would be nice if you could also avoid getting older, since the risk for syndrome X conditions increases with age, but no one has yet figured out how to make that happen!

If you are taking medications for any of the medical conditions you have, take them as instructed. If you are supposed to take your medicine before or after meals, do not wait until bedtime. Certain medications must be timed with body functions in order to be effective. Regular exercise is very important in controlling insulin resistance as well as in reducing your risk for more serious heart disease. Physical exercise affects the tissues and cells of the body in many ways. It stimulates the release of endorphins, natural sub-

stances in your body that cause you to feel good. It stimulates insulin sensitivity in cells, improving their ability to
use insulin and metabolize glucose to give you energy. And
exercise tones and conditions the muscle cells in your arteries and even in your heart, helping them to function more
efficiently and making them less attractive for lipid
deposits.

*I see one doctor for my diabetes and another for my heart
disease. How can I be sure each knows what the other is
doing regarding my treatment?*

It is important for each doctor who is involved in your
care to know what the others are thinking and doing. Particularly with syndromes, what one does affects the conditions
others are trying to treat. Not knowing of other conditions
and treatments could result in one doctor's treatment can-
celing out another, or could even cause harm. Fortunately
for syndrome X conditions, some aspects of treatment are
fundamental to all—namely, weight control, nutrition, and
exercise. Medications to increase insulin sensitivity also
generally have a positive affect on all conditions, because
insulin resistance is at the core of the syndrome.

One way you can help your doctors stay informed about
what each is doing is to request each doctor to send copies
of the record of your office visit to the other doctors immediately following each visit. This way, each medical record
in each doctor's office has a complete picture of your health.
Doctors who are specialists focus on the medical problems
that fall within the realm of their specialties. Though they
are interested in your overall health and well-being, they are
trained to treat a particular kind of problem. This is where
their expertise and skill lies, and they may not be attuned to
other medical concerns that are outside their specialty areas.

Each doctor you see should know what other doctors you
are also seeing, and what conditions they are treating. Then,
with your permission, they can discuss any problems or concerns that arise to arrive at the best medical solution. It does

not hurt to keep a journal for yourself as well, noting when you had an office visit, with which doctor, and what the doctor said and did. You can take this informal record with you to an appointment with a new doctor, or use it to keep track of your progress and any complications or setbacks.

It is not me but a family member who has several syndrome X conditions. How do I help and support my loved one?

One of the most effective things you can do for someone else who has conditions in the syndrome X constellation is to join him or her in the lifestyle changes that are so essential in getting control of these conditions. It is rare that only one person in a household has less than nutritious eating habits and does not exercise. Share in nutritious meals and in physical activities as much as possible. In addition to a good workout, taking walks together can give you time to talk with each other, a rare commodity in today's hectic lifestyle. You might join a gym or health club together, or take up activities you both enjoy, such as bicycling, hiking, or swimming.

My loved one knows he or she has potentially serious health problems, but acts as though nothing is wrong. What can I do?

Unfortunately, you cannot take control of someone else's lifestyle and health. Your loved one must make the necessary changes in order to see his or her health situation improve. As much as possible, be supportive without nagging. This can be a tough balancing act. Lifestyle changes are usually the most difficult aspect of treatment for most people. There is sometimes a sense of guilt or self-blame about being overweight or not exercising or eating junk food. Trying to make changes in these behaviors may force a confrontation with this guilt.

The best way to deal with this is to focus on the future, not the past. Recognize and accept that you cannot change what has already happened. You cannot take back 10 or 20 years of fast food and inactivity. All you can do is change these behaviors in the here and now. Doing so gives you the ability to consciously influence and shape your future health. (Failing to make the necessary changes does so as well.) Other people are angry and resentful that they have medical problems, and resist making any changes they feel are being imposed upon them by forces they cannot control (doctors, symptoms, even you).

You might try making the lifestyle changes yourself that your loved one is resisting. Sometimes seeing someone else make them demonstrates that the changes are not really that bad. It also establishes these new behaviors as the new standard in your household. It is very difficult to do everything in two different ways—to fix two different meals, have two different ways to relax after dinner, and so on. If there are other family members living in your household, involve them in the new behaviors. Even if your loved one continues to resist, the rest of you will enjoy the benefits of the changes.

Some larger communities, particularly those with medical school clinics and hospitals, have support groups for people with diabetes, hypertension, dyslipidemia, PCOS, and even syndrome X. Some support groups are for both those who have these conditions and their family members, while others are for one or the other. If there is no support group in your community, ask your doctor if there would be any interest among his or her patients in getting a support group started.

Increasingly, the Internet provides a way to connect with others who share your concerns and experiences. While it is important to use caution in sharing personal information with strangers, online chat rooms and e-mail forums can provide both knowledge and support. Always check with your doctor about any medical advice you receive from an Internet source. As wonderful as the Internet is, it is also filled with misinformation. Try to identify reliable sources, and stay away from those that tout miracle cures.

7

Natural Remedies and Treatment Alternatives

Most people recognize that conventional medicine, for all of its wonders, has its limitations. People with chronic health conditions often want to do as much as they can to improve their health and well-being. Many look to herbal and natural remedies and treatment alternatives to supplement or even replace conventional medical care. Health risks can be associated with both, depending on the method and the seriousness of the health conditions.

The most important aspect of considering natural remedies and treatment alternatives is knowledge. Learn as much as you can about both the conventional treatments your doctor recommends and the alternative approaches that appeal to you so you can make fully informed decisions. In many situations, the two can safely coexist—as long as your doctor knows what other substances you might be taking, such as herbal preparations. Just because a product is made from herbs does not mean it is inherently safe. There are thousands of toxic plants, many of which have therapeutic value in limited doses but can cause death in higher quantities. On the other hand, there are seldom any conflicts between conventional medical treatment and techniques such as yoga and meditation, which indeed may have many health benefits.

Are there "natural" substances I can substitute for the drugs my doctor wants me to take?

Many medications are in fact derived from natural substances, or synthesized to replicate natural substances. Insulin is a good example. There is often a perception that there is something unnatural about taking prescription medications. What most people mean when they say "natural" is something they do not have to consider medicine, or that is foreign to their bodies. Most of the time, unfortunately, there are no such substances that have the same therapeutic effects as prescription medications. Medications are designed to assist with conditions that result from the natural processes of your body somehow going awry.

The conditions of syndrome X can have mild to serious symptoms. Prompt and appropriate treatment can keep mild problems from becoming serious. Some serious symptoms will almost certainly require aggressive medical intervention to keep them from becoming life-threatening, such as hypertension (which can cause a stroke) and cardiovascular disease (which can cause a heart attack).

Others may have irreversible consequences, such as diabetes, which can cause progressive eye damage resulting in partial to complete blindness (diabetic retinopathy) or kidney damage resulting in the need for dialysis or transplant (renal failure). Such complications are most often the consequence of no or inadequate treatment. The goal of medical treatment is to keep these serious medical problems at bay.

Some people feel they have failed in some way if they develop health conditions that require regular medical care. This is especially likely with conditions where lifestyle factors play a role. If only you had eaten nutritiously and exercised regularly all those years . . . Well, "if only" is an endless game that has no winners. Indeed, your health habits years ago may well have set the stage for your health concerns today. But give yourself a break. We did not know 20 or 30 years ago what we know today about how diet and physical activity affect conditions like diabetes and heart disease. We still do not know the full story, though we do know the connection is strong. We now also know there are other factors involved, too, such as genetics (heredity) and environment (exposure to chemicals and substances such as cigarette smoke).

What matters from this point forward is that you use the knowledge you have gained about your condition to make positive health choices. You know diet and exercise matter, so do the best you can to make the changes you need to make. If your doctor prescribes medication, this is to improve your health and your life. Yes, medications can cause changes in your body that would not happen otherwise. This is not necessarily unnatural. It was not so long ago that people died young from conditions we are today fortunate enough to complain about as mere inconveniences.

Most doctors not only want but also expect their patients to take active responsibility for their health. They do not view the care they provide as an issue of control. They have a particular expertise acquired through study and practice, and they want to use that expertise to help you make informed choices about your health and your medical care. You should feel comfortable discussing your preferences and concerns with your doctor. You should feel confident that your doctor considers your individual circumstances and perspectives when making treatment recommendations. And you should feel like a partner in your health care. One of the most natural things you can do for your health is to take care of your body. It needs nutritious food, adequate rest, and regular exercise.

WARNING: CONSULT YOUR DOCTOR BEFORE MAKING ANY MEDICATION CHANGES

Many medications take time to reach therapeutic levels in your bloodstream and in your tissues. Suddenly changing the dose or stopping the medication could result in undesired side effects and even medical problems. This is especially a concern with many antihypertensives (medications to treat high blood pressure). Suddenly stopping these medications could cause your blood pressure to shoot up in somewhat of a rebound effect. If you have coronary artery disease or cerebrovascular disease, this surge could cause a stroke or even a heart attack. Other medications may also need to be tapered off if you can stop taking them.

Many herbal preparations are promoted as helping a broad range of health conditions. Often, the active ingredients, and thus the actions of these preparations, are not clear. Other herbal remedies target specific conditions. These may have more concentrated ingredients, though again this is not always clear. Sometimes it is this "unknown" that is of greatest concern. Other times, the ingredients in particular herbal remedies are known to interfere or interact with other substances. They may potentiate each other (intensify each other's effects) or counteract one another (cancel each other out). If you are taking prescription medications, you should consult with your doctor before you start taking herbal or natural preparations. If you have been taking herbal preparations, tell your doctor what you take, how much of it you take, and when you take it. It is important to do this *before* your doctor writes out your prescriptions. Your doctor may decide to go with different medications than those originally considered or may suggest changes in your herbal remedies.

CHOOSING SAFE AND EFFECTIVE ALTERNATIVES

The challenge with many herbal and natural preparations is that they have not gone through the rigorous testing and evaluation procedures that drugs must go through. This makes it difficult to say with certainty that a particular product does—or does not—have therapeutic (healing) properties. A second issue is product consistency. Herbal and natural remedies are considered nutritional or dietary supplements in this country, and as such are not required to comply with the same production standards that medicine manufacturers must follow. With medications, every tablet or vial of the same strength contains precisely the same amount of active and inactive ingredients. Each time you take the medication, you receive precisely the same dose. Manufacturers must also follow strict rules about what can be included in the medication as inactive ingredients ("filler" substances that may give the product shape, color, and consistency). These rules do not apply to preparations considered to be dietary supplements.

Although many companies that produce herbal and natural remedies are committed to quality and consistency in their products, some are less reliable. The actual amount of an herb or other natural substance in a preparation (the active ingredient) may vary, sometimes substantially, from one manufacturing lot to another. This makes the product's strength or potency inconsistent and unpredictable. The product you buy this week could be half again as powerful as the product from the same manufacturer that you bought last month. Some would argue that this matters little anyway because many herbal products do not do what their advertising suggests. However, if the product could do what its reputation claims, you might not be receiving the dose you think you are to fulfill those claims. If you choose to use herbal products and natural supplements, buy them from a reputable source such as a well-established health food store, and buy name brands you know to be reliable.

BUYER BEWARE!

Herbal and natural preparations are considered food products, not drugs, under federal guidelines. This means they

cannot claim specific health benefits. Consequently, manufacturers must be more creative in establishing connections
between their products and purported health benefits. Often,
manufacturers use testimonials to accomplish this. Advertising material includes letters from satisfied customers, citing
the health improvements they have noticed since taking the
preparation. The problem is, there seldom is any objective
measure of these benefits. The testimonial reports on the
person's observations about his or her own symptoms are
highly subjective. As well, there is no way to identify other
factors that contributed to health improvements. A person
might start taking an herbal remedy that promotes weight
loss, for example, and at the same time follow the diet
guidelines that come with the product. This changes what
and how they eat, which generally does result in weight loss.
It becomes impossible to know which should get the greater
credit, the herbal remedy or the dietary changes.

Sadly, some profiteers out there are only interested in
taking your money. They offer "get well quick" products
and devices that at best do no harm (along with doing no
good) and at worst can create serious health problems for
you. People who have chronic conditions are often particularly vulnerable to such schemes. But that familiar adage
holds true in health care—if it sounds too good to be true,
it probably is. There is no health treatment with a guaranteed outcome. Even the most standard, successful treatments sometimes do not work as expected or produce
unanticipated results. Through diligence regarding lifestyle
habits and medical recommendations (including prescription medications), most people can control their symptoms
and enjoy relatively normal lives. Some will even be able to
stop taking medication, with the doctor's approval. But
there are no miracle cures out there that can do this for you.
(If there were, you can bet your doctor would have you
taking or using them.) Anything that professes to cure is
quackery.

How can I safely reduce my need for medication?

Discuss with your doctor the ways that this might be done. For example, in many situations, if a person loses weight, becomes more active, and eats a healthier diet, the need for certain medications such as those for blood pressure, lipids, even diabetes may be reduced or even eliminated. This is most likely to happen when symptoms are mild and respond favorably to treatment. Again, one of the most important aspects of treatment for the health conditions of syndrome X is lifestyle.

Some people have always eaten nutritiously, exercised regularly, and maintained a normal body weight—and they still develop health problems related to insulin resistance. There is much doctors do not know about the role of genetics and environment beyond lifestyle habits. If you are such a person, you may find medication is the only way to manage your symptoms and your health, at least for now. There are research studies going on all the time, however, bringing new insights and knowledge to the treatment of syndrome X conditions. The more doctors learn about the intricate functions underlying these conditions, the better able they are to tailor treatment approaches to individual circumstances. Chapter 10 discusses in detail the directions of current research and the outlook for future treatment.

Can garlic lower my cholesterol?

People have used garlic for medicinal purposes for hundreds of years. However, there are no conclusive scientific studies that demonstrate precisely what this herb can do. Some evidence indicates that the active chemical ingredient in garlic, allicin, can lower blood cholesterol levels as well as blood pressure, and might also lower blood sugar levels. These effects are difficult to assess scientifically because some people take garlic supplements while others get their daily dose directly from garlic cloves. Diet and exercise are probably more likely to affect cholesterol and other blood lipids.

At the very least, garlic does appear to help with problems of indigestion, such as bloating and gas, though too much garlic can cause such problems. Some people also take garlic as an antioxidant (a substance believed to boost the body's immune functions). Most garlic preparations contain natural substances that neutralize the herb's distinctive odor.

Can vitamin and mineral supplements improve my syndrome X conditions and my health?

Professionals disagree about how helpful vitamin and mineral supplements are to health in general and to particular medical conditions. Certain vitamin and mineral deficiencies can cause or contribute to medical problems. A lack of vitamin C, for example, causes scurvy (bleeding into body tissues and poor healing), and a lack of vitamin D causes rickets (bone deformities). Not enough of the B vitamins can cause megaloblastic anemia (low hemoglobin in the blood). These conditions can occur in people with serious chronic illnesses who do not eat well, and as a result of various disorders that interfere with the body's ability to absorb nutrients. Some medications can cause mild vitamin deficiencies by interfering with vitamin absorption and use. This is a possible side effect of some lipid-lowering drugs, for example. Such situations are treated with vitamin and mineral supplements to restore the body's normal levels of these vital substances.

Vitamin and mineral supplements are also helpful when your diet does not contain the nutrients your body needs. A good example of this is calcium. Most women and many men do not get enough calcium through food sources. Dairy products are the most common source of calcium, but many people who are watching their fat intake tend to cut dairy products entirely out of their diets rather than switching to low-fat products. Calcium supplements help replace dietary calcium, though there are some questions as to whether this fully meets the body's needs. Calcium citrate is most easily absorbed. The foods that supply vitamins and minerals also provide other substances, such as flavonoids and phyto-chemicals, whose roles in nutrition and health are not fully understood but which are abundantly present in many foods. These substances often exist in microscopic quantities, and there are hundreds of them. It is not feasible, and sometimes not possible, to artificially reproduce them to include in sup-plement formulas. Researchers do not yet know what role these substances have. They may potentiate (augment) the actions of certain vitamins and minerals, or have distinct functions of their own.

It is not clear whether taking higher amounts of vitamins and minerals, especially in the form of supplements, to boost the body's levels of them has any beneficial effect. Some doctors believe that magnesium helps diabetes and high blood pressure, and chromium helps diabetes. In indi-vidual cases they may. There just is not any good way to measure the effects of supplements, and good scientific studies are either lacking or confusing.

Some vitamins and minerals can become toxic at high levels, notably vitamins A and E, and minerals such as iron and zinc. Your body excretes excess amounts of water-soluble vitamins (the B-complex and vitamin C), raising ques-tions about the value of taking more than is needed to meet the daily recommended requirements. Vitamins A, D, E, and K are fat-soluble, which means your body stores any excess amounts of them in fat tissue. The advantage of this is that your body can draw from these stores when your dietary intake of these vitamins drops, but the drawback is that they can accumulate to levels that cause health problems.

Some doctors recommend a niacin supplement, (a B vita-min also known as nicotinic acid), for people with lipid dis-orders. Niacin is involved in the body's metabolism of fats and carbohydrates. Some evidence indicates that increasing niacin in the diet, either through eating more foods that con-tain it or through supplements, can decrease blood lipid lev-els. It appears to improve the functioning of the enzymes involved in metabolism. Niacin can have a number of side effects, including interference with some medications (such as cholesterol-lowering drugs) and glucose levels. Talk with your doctor before taking niacin.

I have heard that certain foods can help various medical problems. What foods can help syndrome X conditions?

As this book stresses, a nutritious diet is an essential component of treating syndrome X conditions. Health experts generally recommend going lighter on the carbohydrates and fats, though they do not suggest you try to eliminate these substances because doing so deprives your body of nutrients that it needs. (See Chapters 8 and 9 for more about diet recommendations, fad diets, and eating habits.) Beyond a generally nutritious diet, there do seem to be certain foods that help and others that hinder the conditions of syndrome X. A diet very low in fat, such as a vegan diet (strict vegetarian diet that allows no animal products), can halt and even reverse certain forms of heart disease in some people. The program developed by physician Dean Ornish (discussed later in this chapter) incorporates such a diet with other elements including exercise and stress reduction. Despite the benefits, it is often difficult for people to follow such a strict diet.

FOODS THAT HELP

Ancient Egyptian physicians prescribed a diet high in wheat grains for diabetes. Ancient Chinese healers recommended ginseng, while their Middle East counterparts suggested raw onions and garlic. As it turns out, these foods contain chemicals that can lower blood sugar levels and even improve insulin sensitivity. Onions and garlic, for example, contain allicin, which is closely related chemically to the glucose-lowering drug tolbutamide. These foods do not contain enough of these chemicals to function as the sole treatment for diabetes, of course.

Most doctors do not endorse using such foods in an effort to regulate your insulin and blood sugar levels. If you like onions and garlic, enjoy. But eat a diet that is nutritionally balanced and get regular physical exercise. This is the surest way to maintain your body's health.

Oat bran and oatmeal gained popularity in the 1980s as a food capable of improving blood cholesterol levels (lowering LDL or "bad" cholesterol and raising HDL or "good" cholesterol). Whole grain oats contain water-soluble fiber that binds with cholesterol and other lipids in the intestines, partially blocking these fatty substances from being absorbed into the bloodstream. Other foods that appear to also contain lipid-fighting substances are legumes such as beans (pinto, navy, kidney, black, and soy). Raw fruits and vegetables that are high in fiber are also helpful.

In the spotlight for its ability to influence blood sugar and insulin levels is broccoli. This unassuming vegetable has ten times as much of a trace mineral called chromium as any other food. Chromium appears to enhance the function of insulin, making it more effective in lowering blood sugar. Barley, mushrooms, nuts, oysters, and rhubarb are other foods that contain chromium. Because the typical American diet is high in fats and carbohydrates and relatively low in other nutrients, health experts estimate that most Americans do not get enough chromium. Some believe this is a key reason for the steady rise in the number of cases of type 2 diabetes, but this is far from proven.

FOODS THAT HINDER

Most people now understand that excess fat in the foods they eat becomes excess fat in their bodies. The connection between saturated fat and high cholesterol is undeniable. But dietary fat is a significant factor in diabetes, too. A diet high in fat seems to reduce cell sensitivity to insulin. Too much of foods such as potatoes can be a problem in diabetes as well. Potatoes are high in complex carbohydrates (starches), which for many years doctors believed were "safer" than simple carbohydrates such as are common in candy. Research in the 1980s challenged this belief when it demonstrated that blood sugar levels rise more rapidly after eating foods such as potatoes and white rice than after eating candy. Complex carbohydrates become sugar in your body relatively quickly, but are also used quickly for energy. This research gave birth to the food glycemic index, a scale for measuring how quickly foods cause blood sugar to rise (more on this in Chapter 9).

Many foods have a compound effect. A baked potato topped with butter, sour cream, and bacon bits can hit your metabolism like a hand grenade, exploding both your blood lipid levels and your blood sugar levels. It does not usually serve you well to attempt to eliminate certain kinds of foods from your diet, however. Your body needs a wide range of nutrients, and depriving it of selective ones can create an entirely different set of health problems.

THE ORNISH PROGRAM

An American medical doctor, Dean Ornish, developed a very strict regimen that appears to stop and even reverse heart disease in people who are willing to adhere to its requirements. The Ornish program contains four key elements: a vegan diet that is less than 10% fat, moderate daily exercise, individual and group therapy, and stress-reduction techniques such as meditation, yoga, and tai chi.

In very controlled groups, the Ornish program has had impressive success in halting the progress of heart disease. In some people, the program seems to even turn back the clock, restoring the person's body to an even healthier state. The program's success has been so impressive, in fact, that in 1999 the federal government decided to authorize Medicare funds to cover the costs of the program for Medicare participants who want to try the rather unorthodox approach. Researchers plan to study the results to see how effective the Ornish program can be with a wider base of patients.

A unique aspect of the program is its integration of body and mind in the healing process. The key to the success of the Ornish program is the absolute compliance of participants with the program's requirements, which really represent a total lifestyle shift. Because of the extreme nature of the Ornish program, it is not for everyone. A person must be wholly committed to all aspects of the program, and willing to maintain them for life.

Can relaxation techniques help lower my blood pressure or improve other aspects of my health?

Relaxation techniques are often helpful in chronic health conditions. A common criticism of Western medicine is that it focuses on diseases and problems without regard for their relationships to each other or to the rest of a person's whole being—physical, emotional, and spiritual. Many relaxation techniques attempt to reconnect these elements to focus on the whole person. This is sometimes called the mind-body connection. It is an approach that acknowledges and respects the power of the mind and the spirit to affect the physical body. Some people refer to this as a positive attitude.

From a scientific perspective, relaxation techniques achieve mixed results. While many people report feeling better after practicing them, there are few studies that have been able to document consistent, repeatable outcomes. This is the standard by which we measure a treatment's effectiveness in this country. There are studies that have demonstrated consistent drops in blood pressure when study participants regularly practice certain relaxation techniques such as meditation. Some medical centers now incorporate meditation as well as visualization in preoperative and postoperative care for people undergoing major surgery. They have found that people who can envision themselves as well tend to heal more quickly, as do those who can achieve a sense of inner calm through meditation or prayer. These are not approaches that replace conventional medical care, but that supplement or augment it.

VISUALIZATION

Do you ever sit in front of your computer while you are at work, or stand in a long line and find that your mind has wandered to a different place and time? Perhaps you are remembering a vacation to Hawaii, or anticipating a week-end in the mountains. When this happens at random, we call it daydreaming. When you can intentionally direct your mind to take you somewhere else, we call it visualization. Athletes and musicians frequently use visualization to pre-pare for events and performances, for example. They picture themselves making the big play or hitting the high notes with ease and perfection, and they play this mental movie over and over in their minds until it is the only way they can see themselves. Instead of letting their minds drift to what might go wrong, which is a natural direction for unchan-neled thoughts to take, they see themselves doing everything right. Coaches and conductors are convinced it is a tech-nique that makes a difference.

Many people are convinced it is a technique that can make a difference in your health, too. Experts in visualization sug-gest that you start by taking a comfortable position in a place where you feel safe and protected. You might sit in a favorite chair or lie on your bed (as long as you do not go to sleep!). Close your eyes, and try to envision your health condition. If you have diabetes, maybe you try to see your cells sur-rounded by insulin and sugar particles. You see the cells ignoring the insulin, and the sugar particles building up as the insulin fails to usher them into the cells where they can become metabolized for fuel. Then concentrate on seeing a swarm of friendly helpers appear—the chemicals from your insulin-sensitizing medication have arrived. They encourage your cells to open up to allow more insulin through, carrying more sugar inside. Envision the happy process of metabolism, and the sugar particles gradually diminishing. See your cells become satisfied as they receive the nourishment they need and your body achieves balance.

Such a visualization exercise does not actually cause these events to occur, of course (at least not as far as science is able to determine), and you are certainly free to envision a different scenario. But the process of visualization does make you very conscious of what is going on inside your body. It helps you focus on what can go right rather than what is wrong. Doctors will be the first to tell you that many things happen in sickness and in health that defy explanation. Having a positive vision of your own wellness certainly cannot hurt anything. Just be sure you also continue to follow your doctor's treatment recommendations.

MEDITATION

Meditation is a way to calm the mind, and correspondingly, the body. A common misperception about meditation is that it is an intense, spiritual experience in which your mind enters an altered state of consciousness. Though certain forms of meditation can indeed be deep and trancelike, more commonly meditation is a process of consciously focusing your thoughts in a directed fashion. There are many forms of meditation that do this in different ways. The goal is to achieve a sense of inner calm and to release emotional stress. For many people, prayer is a form of meditation. Meditation is particularly effective for many people because you can do it any time, anywhere.

BIOFEEDBACK

Researchers have studied biofeedback as a way to affect a variety of conditions known to have some component of stress involved, such as migraine headaches and chronic pain. Some people are able to use biofeedback to affect their symptoms. Others have been able to affect what are traditionally viewed as involuntary body functions such as pulse and blood pressure.

Biofeedback involves using monitoring equipment to measure the particular function, such as blood pressure. Over time, the person sees certain patterns that correlate to certain activities or feelings of stress. By using various relaxation techniques, the person learns to cause changes in those patterns, reflecting an effect on the function. Eventually the person will be able to cause changes at will through relaxation techniques, and does not need to use the monitoring equipment. Biofeedback is not effective for many people, and may not have any effect on conditions such as certain kinds of hypertension that have primarily physiological causes. It takes a great deal of time and commitment to use biofeedback successfully.

YOGA

Yoga is sometimes called the perfect activity, because it exercises both the body and the mind. Many yoga movements emphasize awareness and control, both physical and mental. These movements can be so simple that you can do them anywhere, or complex enough to require considerable practice (and guidance from a yoga instructor).

People who are unfamiliar with the concepts and practices of yoga often view this ancient form of exercise as a collection of body contortions only the double-jointed can perform. Though advanced postures do require skill and flexibility, nearly everyone can do at least the basic postures and breathing techniques. Eastern philosophy puts the focus of yoga on controlling the energy of your body, mind, and spirit to achieve balance. It does so by combining breathing techniques with postures that open or release various energy channels. These breathing techniques are essential to yoga, since traditional yoga philosophy measures life in terms of breaths, not time. From a Western perspective, yoga stretches, tones, and relaxes muscle groups. The breathing techniques clear your mind of distracting thoughts, allowing you to feel a sense of inner harmony. They also enhance your lung capacity, enabling you to draw more oxygen into your system with each breath you take.

Yoga has become quite popular in our fast-paced culture because it offers the opportunity to stop rushing around and just "be" for a brief period of time. Though yoga is not considered an aerobic activity (exercise that increases your heart rate and breathing), a well-rounded session can leave you feeling like you have had a vigorous workout. Yoga is also popular because it does not require special clothing, equipment, or facilities. Most people report feeling rested and relaxed following a yoga session. The best way to learn yoga is to take classes so you can see how the postures are done and have an experienced yogi (yoga master) teach you to do them correctly. You can hurt yourself doing yoga if you attempt postures beyond your ability or perform postures incorrectly.

Yoga breathing techniques, which you can do as simple movements or as the basis for more complex movements, are great for relieving stress and helping you to regain a sense of control in particularly stressful times. Basic yoga breathing techniques are easy to learn, and you can do them just about anywhere without drawing attention to yourself. The simplest of these is called "alternate nostril breathing."

To do this technique, sit comfortably but with your spine straight and your chin level. Hold one nostril shut, and take a slow, deep breath in through the open nostril. Fill your lungs, and then hold the breath there for a count of five.

Switch nostrils and slowly breathe out, letting your lungs empty. Repeat the technique until you feel your muscles and your mind relax. The key is to breathe slowly and deeply. Many people close their eyes and focus on envisioning life-giving oxygen entering their lungs and their bodies, and the toxins of metabolism and stress leaving.

TAI CHI

Tai chi is a form of ancient Eastern martial arts. Unlike the more familiar forms of karate and judo, which feature quick, powerful moves, tai chi incorporates a blend of structured movements, breathing techniques, and meditation. Movements are slow and deliberate, and may involve holding a posture for several minutes before gradually transitioning to the next movement. Tai chi can be done in groups or individually, and often looks like a combination of yoga and dance. The physical movements are excellent for maintaining muscle tone and strength as well as for improving balance. The breathing techniques and meditation components of tai chi leave participants feeling relaxed and at peace after a session. People who regularly practice tai chi often find that this sense of relaxation lasts up to several hours after the tai chi session ends. Many community centers and health clubs offer classes in tai chi.

What about antioxidants?

Antioxidants are natural substances that attack molecules called free radicals. These molecules are missing electrons, making them unstable. They attempt to stabilize themselves by taking the electrons they need from other complete molecules, which then destabilizes those molecules. This process is called oxidation, and sets in action a chain of events that results in cell and tissue damage and ultimately disease. Many research studies are attempting to more fully understand the role and significance of oxidation, as well as ways to combat it. Substances such as vitamin E, vitamin C, beta carotene, and the mineral selenium have gotten much attention as antioxidants. They appear to interfere with the robbery attempts of free radicals, attacking and destroying these incomplete molecules before they can do damage. Many health experts recommend a diet high in foods that are natural sources of antioxidants, such as fresh fruits and vegetables (the fresher the better). Though many people take supplements that contain antioxidants, it is not clear whether these have the same effect. Literally thousands of the chemical substances in natural foods are impossible to synthesize in supplements, and researchers do not yet know how significant they are in supporting the actions of antioxidants.

Can ginkgo biloba improve my circulation?

Some evidence indicates that regularly taking the herb ginkgo biloba improves circulation particularly in the brain, which aids in memory and concentration. Ginkgo biloba may even delay the onset of Alzheimer's disease, a disabling and progressive disorder in which brain cells degenerate, according to a landmark study reported in the *Journal of the American Medical Association* in 1997. It appears that ginkgo biloba has a mild anticoagulating effect. That is, it works as a mild blood "thinner" to keep platelets from sticking to one another. It also appears to have some effect on the fatty accumulations that can build up inside the arteries.

Do not take ginkgo biloba if you are taking prescription anticoagulants (blood thinners) or aspirin. Doing so can increase the anticoagulation effect, making you susceptible to easy bleeding and poor clotting. Common anticoagulant medications include dicoumarol and warfarin (marketed under numerous brand names). Many doctors, as well as the American Heart Association, recommend an aspirin a day a for the drug's mild anticoagulant effect to reduce the risk of heart attack.

Are there herbal or natural remedies that could be harmful?

Any substance you take has the potential to be harmful. Because herbal and "natural" preparations are considered food products rather than drugs, they can contain a wide variety of ingredients that, were those ingredients present in a drug, would be considered impurities. This is one risk with such preparations. Another potential problem with herbal and natural remedies is the possibility that they could interact with each other or with medications you are also taking.

People tend to believe products that are "natural" are safer than manufactured products. This is not true. There are many poisonous substances that occur in nature, some of which, under very controlled use, can have therapeutic effects. One example is digitalis, a powerful chemical found in the leaves and stems of the foxglove plant. Ancient healers often used tea brewed from foxglove leaves to aid their patients with heart failure. Ancient medical texts document that drinking a cup of this tea concoction, prepared to precise specifications, every day could keep the heart beating strong for many years. The margin of safety for digitalis is very slim, however, and it does not take much beyond the therapeutic dose to bring an abrupt end to life, which ancient medical texts also documented. (Today doctors prescribe medications, synthesized in laboratories, that mimic the active ingredients of digitalis, and monitor blood levels regularly to be sure the dose remains at a therapeutic level.) While the line between life and death is not so fine with most herbal and natural preparations on the market today, nearly all have potentially dangerous side effects if taken in high doses.

Some herbal products that promote weight loss contain stimulants such as ephedrine (sometimes identified in the list of ingredients as ephedra) and caffeine. Ephedrine is a member of the same chemical family as amphetamine but is not as strong. Other medicinal products, such as over-the-counter diet preparations and cold medicines, contain caffeine and ephedrine or similar substances. Caffeine is perhaps one of the most common stimulants, appearing in products ranging from coffee and tea to some soft drinks and chocolate.

Stimulants often work as appetite suppressants—people feel less hungry when they take them. But stimulants also rev up the heart and the nervous system. They raise blood pressure and the pulse rate. They also stimulate the brain to release endorphins, which can produce a mild "high" or sense of euphoria. Caffeine causes blood vessels to dilate, or widen, allowing a higher volume of blood to pass through them. These effects can be dangerous. In someone with cardiovascular disease or hypertension, the sudden surge in blood pressure, pulse, and blood volume can trigger a potentially fatal heart attack or stroke. Too much caffeine can cause heart palpitations, the sensation that your heart is fluttering.

Another risk with herbal and natural remedies is that people who take them sometimes stop taking medications prescribed by their doctors, or treat themselves without ever seeing a doctor. This can permit health conditions that are easily treatable in their early stages to develop into serious problems requiring aggressive medical intervention, such as heart disease, kidney disease, and eye problems, including blindness.

Do I have to tell my doctor I'm taking herbal or natural substances?

Some people worry that their doctors will disapprove of them "going around" the doctor to try other healing methods on their own. This is not usually the issue. Most doctors encourage their patients to take responsibility for their health and wellness. However, they want their patients to talk with them about any alternative therapies they are considering. This is because such therapies may have an effect on the treatment the doctor has already prescribed. Sometimes the doctor can make adjustments in the allopathic treatment (conventional medical care) to accommodate alternative therapies. Sometimes alternative therapies are not appropriate for an individual's situation, and the doctor can provide explanations and information about why. Some doctors do disapprove of herbal or natural remedies, because these often have not been studied in the same comprehensive, rigorous manner in which drugs and medications are studied. For this reason, there is no proof of their effectiveness. Some natural and herbal remedies are actually harmful.

Despite any concerns you have about your doctor's feelings toward natural and herbal remedies, it is essential for you to tell your doctor about any that you are taking or considering. This includes herbal teas, which many people tend to think of as soothing beverages rather than substances that can affect body functions. Herbal teas can contain medicinal ingredients, however. Chamomile tea, for example, contains chemicals that relax muscle tissues. Indeed, your doctor might even recommend chamomile tea for its ability to soothe digestive upsets.

Herbal and natural products sometimes contain substances that interact with drugs your doctor has prescribed, or that in some way affect metabolism. These remedies can interfere with other treatment. Ginseng, for example, is a common herbal remedy used to increase energy. It does this by acting as a stimulant within your body. But ginseng also stimulates your body to produce testosterone—definitely not a desired action for women in general and particularly for women who have PCOS. It is also crucial for you to tell any doctor who might perform surgery on you of any herbal or natural remedies you are using, even if you use them just occasionally. Many of these substances are known to interact with the drugs commonly used during anesthesia and can result in a nasty drug interaction problem for you.

How can I find out more about vitamins and natural remedies?

When it comes to information about vitamins and natural remedies, there's certainly no shortage. It seems that seldom does a week go by without reports of new research findings. In an effort to help people sort through the myriad of studies, reports, and claims, the National Institutes of Health (NIH) has established the National Center for Complementary and Alternative Medicine (NCCAM) to function as a clearinghouse for information about complementary medicine and natural alternatives. The "Resources and Additional Information" section at the end of this book tells you how to contact the NCCAM.

8

*

Taking Care of Yourself:
Weight Control

Many health experts believe obesity is the number one health problem confronting the United States today. More than 97 million people in this country are overweight—more than half the population. Nearly 45 million are obese—one in four Americans. The reasons for the steady rise in excess weight are complex and intertwined. People living in this country today enjoy a standard of living like no other generation before them. Fast food is in, and intense physical activity—work-related or recreational—is out. And weight is up. The situation alarms health experts. Obesity can shave years from a person's life expectancy. Factor in the myriad of health problems that typically coexist with obesity by middle age, and we are looking at one of history's most lethal killers. Obesity and the health conditions linked to it are expensive as well, costing $70 billion a year for health care services.

Obesity and overweight are key features of syndrome X as well, affecting the majority of people with its conditions. There appears to be a clear relationship between excess body fat and insulin resistance—the more fat tissue, the less sensitive to insulin the body's cells become. Many of the symptoms of syndrome X conditions improve with weight loss as the amount of fat tissue diminishes.

What is overweight?

Overweight is an increase in the adipose, or fat, tissue in the body. A more accurate term would be "overfat," because the issue is not so much weight as it is the percentage of that weight that is body fat. People who are overweight weigh up to 20% more than normal. Traditionally, overweight has been determined by body weight as measured with a scale, with norms established according to height. Today, doctors use a more precise measurement called the body mass index (BMI), which presents a mathematical relationship between weight and height. Many doctors also include waist size when attempting to determine whether a person who weighs more than the norm is overfat. Overweight is a health problem because it is associated with numerous health conditions.

What is obesity?

Obesity is a more serious form of overweight. People who are obese are more than 30% overweight. *Morbid or medical obesity* is the most severe form of obesity in which the obesity threatens the person's life. Like overweight, obesity is measured by BMI.

What causes obesity?

Obesity is a complex medical condition. Doctors do not fully understand all the mechanisms that contribute to its development. In the most simplistic view, obesity results when you consistently eat more food than your body needs to use as fuel. This points to lifestyle factors such as eating and exercise habits. However, there is increasing evidence that genetic factors may play a significant role in whether a person becomes obese. Some research points to enzymes in the body and other biochemical processes that influence various aspects of metabolism. Other research focuses on hereditary predisposition, looking for explanations for why obesity appears to run in families. There are also various emotional factors that influence why people overeat.

THE THRIFTY GENE THEORY AND OTHER HEREDITARY INFLUENCES

Everyone knows people who seem able to eat whatever they want and still stay skinny as a fence post. And everyone knows someone who is constantly dieting, yet never seems to lose weight (or continues to gain). Nor has it escaped notice that in some families nearly all family members are obese, a pattern that often extends through several generations. It is as though some people are born to be thin, and others are born to be fat. This has fueled the search for genetic or hereditary factors that might establish a predisposition toward obesity.

One direction this search has taken is called the thrifty gene theory, sometimes called selective insulin resistance. This theory holds that once upon a time, when people were primarily hunters and gathers, food supplies were alternately abundant and scarce. To survive, they needed the ability to make it through the sometimes extended periods when food was not available. So the bodies of these early people were genetically encoded to be able to store large amounts of fat to sustain them. Researchers believe this encoding has remained, even though people no longer need it. In today's environment, where food is plentiful, this genetic programming continues to run, establishing the foundation for insulin resistance as a health problem rather than a survival attribute. Though the specific genes accountable for this function have not been identified, most researchers accept this theory as a valid explanation for why people of European descent—whose distant ancestors had the need to survive for weeks or even months with little or no food—seem to convert glucose to fat more easily.

Other research has uncovered specific genes that affect obesity. Mutations in these genes appear to contribute to obesity and related conditions such as diabetes by influencing metabolism. Some researchers believe the mutated genes interfere with the enzymes that are involved in the insulin-glucose interactions. Others believe the interference is instead with the signals between fat tissue in the body and the parts of the brain that regulate how the body stores fat. One important point to keep in mind when evaluating the role of heredity in obesity is that genetic predisposition is an influence, not an inevitability. It is one of numerous factors that contribute to obesity. Though researchers have identified genes that affect obesity, they do not fully understand how they do so, or what potential therapeutic value the knowledge holds.

THE SET POINT THEORY

The set point theory holds that each person is "preprogrammed" to have a certain level of body fat. The body will continue storing fat until this set point is reached, much as a room's temperature wants to stay at the thermostat's set point. The person may gain and lose weight over his or her lifetime, but the body will attempt to stay close to its set point. This theory is popular, though it does not have a lot of scientific evidence to support it. A number of processes within the body affect weight and fat regulation—insulin and glucose, of course, as well as neuropeptides, opoids, and alpha and beta adrenergics. Their interactions with each other and various body systems are intricate and probably interconnected, making it difficult to assess how each influences fat storage, metabolism, and obesity. Those who support the set point theory point to the number of people who, no matter how many pounds they lose, ultimately return to the same weight. Others note that many people do lose weight and keep it off, implying that if there is a set point, it can be reset by changing exercise and eating habits.

ENVIRONMENT AND HABIT

Most researchers believe that environment and habit are significant factors in obesity, whether or not there are genetic connections. The majority of people who are overweight or obese do not get much physical activity. Nor do they eat as nutritiously as health guidelines recommend. Sometimes the culprit is lack of information about what foods are healthy and beneficial, and what foods can be detrimental. While knowledge about the roles of diet and nutrition in health and disease has grown tremendously over the past 30 years or so, eating habits have not kept pace. Many people follow eating patterns established several generations ago, when everyday life was hard, physical work. Today's culture is vastly different. Most people sit or stand in one place all day, operating machinery that now does the work. They no longer need a large intake of carbohydrate and fat, though they are still getting it. They eat a lot of food because their families have always eaten a lot of food. Unless they also burn a lot of calories through physical activity, the food on the plate becomes fat in the body.

Studies show that physical activity habits tend to run in families too, though as a function of habit rather than heredity. People whose parents engaged in regular exercise of some sort—swimming, hiking, horseback riding, tennis, bicycling, organized sports such as softball, or even just walking—are more likely to also incorporate physical activity into their adult lives. The reverse seems to be true as well. These are not absolutes, of course, which is part of what makes the heredity versus environment exploration so challenging.

INFLUENCES OF SOCIETY AND CULTURE

Until the twentieth century, it was a sign of affluence to be overweight. A rotund figure conveyed the message that you had more than enough to eat and did not have to engage in menial physical labor. People who worked long, hard hours every day and had little to eat were lean and even gaunt. The advent of the industrial age changed this. Instead of going to work every day to shovel coal or walk behind a horse-drawn plow, people began operating machines that took over such tasks. Work became less physically intense. Correspondingly, improvements in wages and working hours left people with more money and leisure time. They could buy enough food to eat themselves into corpulence, then lounge around enjoying their newfound comfort. Today, food is not only plentiful but also fast. Leisure time is at a historic high. The combination has boosted body weight to new levels too.

PSYCHOLOGICAL AND EMOTIONAL ASPECTS

For many people, food is comfort. Eating satisfies emotional needs as well as (and often instead of) physical hunger. This can become a health problem when it leads to overeating that results in obesity. Sometimes the underlying issues are deep-seated and will require the abilities of a qualified therapist or counselor to unravel them.

Until these issues are resolved, they can interfere with efforts to make lifestyle changes. People who are overweight or obese often feel unaccepted in contemporary society, which seems to worship thinness even though people who are at or below their ideal weights are in the minority. Social factors sometimes influence people who are overweight to delay seeking medical attention for health problems and to feel guilty for having health problems.

How does exercise influence obesity?

Exercise increases your metabolism, or the rate at which you burn calories. It also improves insulin sensitivity, allowing your cells to use glucose more efficiently. With regular exercise, your insulin levels stay lower and your lean body tissue increases. Regular exercise also boosts your resting metabolism, keeping cell activity at a higher level even when your body is at rest. And it builds muscle, which is important, because muscle tissue is more sensitive to the action of insulin than is fat tissue.

An indirect but still important aspect of exercise is that it makes you feel better. Physical activity improves your mood. Some studies indicate that regular moderate exercise, such as brisk walking, can be as effective as medication for treating mild depression.

Why is obesity a health problem?

Obesity is associated with numerous serious health conditions, which doctors call co-morbidities. Though the direct link is not clearly understood, risks for these conditions increase with weight gain and decrease with weight loss.

- **Diabetes**. Obesity and diabetes seem linked through insulin resistance and elevated blood sugar levels. Extra weight decreases insulin sensitivity, while weight loss improves it.
- **Heart disease**. Like diabetes, one link with obesity seems to be insulin resistance. Obesity also puts significant strain on the heart, which must work harder to pump blood through so much extra tissue. This can result in hypertension, cardiovascular disease, and congestive heart failure.
- **Back problems**. Excess body weight puts tremendous strain on the structures of the back, especially when the weight is carried primarily through the abdomen. Abdominal obesity causes a person to stand with the pelvis somewhat tipped forward and the back somewhat arched. This particularly stresses the lumbar region (lower back).
- **Arthritis**. Excess body weight also puts tremendous stress on weight-bearing joints such as the hips,

knees, and ankles. This can cause and subsequently aggravate degenerative arthritis.

- **Other health problems**. Obesity is connected with a wide range of other health problems as well, including gallbladder disease, breathing difficulty, some cancers, and emotional and psychological problems.

Are certain kinds of body fat worse than others?

Certain patterns of body fat distribution correlate more strongly with health problems and diseases. Central, or abdominal, obesity (the "apple" body shape), in which fat accumulates around the belly, is linked to a higher incidence of type 2 diabetes and heart disease than either total body obesity or lower body obesity (the "pear" body shape). Excess fat is probably not good for you no matter where it collects, though.

How is obesity linked to syndrome X?

Obesity is linked to syndrome X through its connections to the conditions of the insulin-resistance syndrome. Obesity is a major risk factor for these conditions.

Can insulin resistance or type 2 diabetes cause obesity?

This has been postulated as one theory attempting to explain the high ratio of overweight and obesity found among people who have type 2 diabetes. Some people have a very difficult time losing weight, leading researchers to explore whether insulin resistance somehow makes an individual more susceptible to weight gain. So far, little evidence supports this theory, and most doctors believe it is the other way around—that excess body weight is a causative factor in insulin resistance and type 2 diabetes. Supporting this belief is consistent evidence that insulin resistance and type 2 diabetes often improve with weight loss.

Doctors believe other factors are at work in people who

do all the right things—eat nutritiously and get plenty of exercise—and still have difficulty losing weight. A genetic predisposition to obesity may interfere with weight loss efforts. Other metabolic disorders could be present, such as hypothyroidism (low thyroid enzymes), which slows metabolism.

How much should I weigh?

For several decades, we have thought about obesity in terms of body weight. There are numerous charts that identify a "normal" range of weight according to height (and sometimes considering whether a person has small, medium, or large bone structure). This system does not actually measure body fat, however, which is really the critical factor. A more accurate way to look at whether you have more body fat than is healthy is by determining your body mass index, or BMI. The BMI uses a formula that roughly calculates what percentage of your body weight is fat. Many health experts consider this to be a more accurate indicator of health because weight itself is not always the issue. People with substantial muscle mass may appear overweight according to just body weight, for example (such as professional athletes), yet have a very low fat-to-muscle ratio.

THE BMI SCALE

The BMI scale uses a mathematical formula to establish a relationship between body weight and height. It is equal to the weight in kilograms divided by height in meters squared, written as $BMI = kg/m^2$. The resulting index, or number, identifies the relative risk of developing certain health problems. The National Institutes of Health categories BMI results in the following manner:

18.5 or less—underweight, with possible health risks
18.6 to 24.9—normal, with average health risks

25.0 to 27.9—overweight, with increased health risks
28.0 to 39.9—obese, with very high health risks
40 or greater—extremely obese, with extremely high
   health risks

HOW TO CALCULATE YOUR BMI

To calculate your BMI:

1. Weigh yourself on an accurate scale (without clothes).
2. Multiply your weight in pounds by .45 (converts it to kilograms).
3. Measure your height (have someone help you so you get a correct measurement), and convert the measurement to inches.
4. Multiply your height in inches by .025 (converts it to meters), then multiply the result by itself (squares it).
5. Divide your weight in kilograms by your height in meters squared.

The result is your BMI. Say, for example, that you weigh 160 pounds and you are 5 feet, 8 inches tall. Multiplied by .45, your weight in kilograms is 72 kg. Your height in inches is 68 inches. Multiplied by .025, your height in meters is 1.7 m. Squared, this is 2.9 m^2. When you divide your weight in kilograms (72) by your height in meters squared (2.9), you get a BMI of 24.8. This is at the high end of normal.

What is the best way to control my weight?
The best way to control your weight is to stop thinking in terms of appearance and image and start thinking in terms of health and wellness. Many people approach weight loss from the perspective of trying to look good for the high

school reunion or a summer vacation on the beach. Though this may get the job done in the short term, what happens once these goals are past? Often, there is no incentive to maintain the weight loss, and the pounds creep back on.

THINK "LIFESTYLE"

Weight loss is not about dieting. It is not really about exercise, either. And it is not really a matter of "loss" so much as "management." Weight management is a matter of lifestyle. It is healthy eating and regular physical activity. Americans are too much in the "diet" mode. We diet, lose weight, stop dieting, go back to our previous habits, and the weight goes back on. Now if you shift into "lifestyle" mode, everything changes. You are no longer so concerned with losing weight to fit into that pair of $150 jeans that has been gathering dust in your closet. Instead, your mission is to lower your BMI to reduce your risk of diabetes, high blood pressure, and heart disease.

Admittedly, this is a tough transition. After all, you see those jeans lying there on the shelf every time you open your closet. The health consequences of diabetes, high blood pressure, and heart disease could be years and even decades away. You have had your entire lifetime to this point to develop the habits that now define your lifestyle. It is no small challenge to start over and replace them. Nonetheless, it is a crucial challenge for you to meet. Start slow, and make steady progress. You will not become a new person overnight—not physically, and not mentally. You are retraining your brain and your thought processes just as you are retraining your body and your taste buds.

It is okay to give yourself little goals for motivation. But reward yourself in positive ways that support your new habits. The old you might have celebrated losing 20 pounds with dinner out and chocolate mousse for dessert. The new you will have to learn how to celebrate dropping ten points on your LDL cholesterol with an apple and an extra 15 minutes tagged onto your daily walk to give the next ten points a good send-off. Practice envisioning yourself as you want to look and feel—healthy and fit—and keep this image with you like a cherished photograph.

And be kind to yourself. If you slip up now and again, that is okay, too. Just get back on track. Did you ever move to a new house that was just a few miles from your old house, then every now and then find yourself driving to the old house on the way home from work? You laugh (maybe swear the third or fourth time it happens), and turn around to go to your new home. Change takes time. Just as you eventually settled into your new routine and your new neighborhood, you will settle into your new habits and your new lifestyle.

GET MOVING!

If there is a magic elixir, it is exercise. Not aerobic dance or weight lifting or basketball, necessarily (though these are wonderful, too), but just ordinary physical activity: walking the dog; taking the stairs instead of the elevator; even swinging in the park when no one is watching. Physical activity feels good. It cheers your body and your mind. And it burns calories, which, as you know, helps send those fat cells packing. It appears that a little activity goes a long way. Several studies have compared people who fidget and move around frequently, even when sitting, to people who are fairly still unless engaged in a specific activity. These studies found that minor but steady level of activity among the fidgeters seemed to make them less likely to gain weight than their nonfidgeting counterparts.

Small activities like parking at the back of the lot instead of looking for a space by the door, walking down the hallway to talk with a coworker rather than calling on the phone, walking to check the mail instead of driving by on your way home from work, and using the stairs instead of the elevator can quickly add up when it comes to using energy. The best thing about these small activities is that they do not require planning or preparation. Your day is filled with dozens of opportunities to get a little bit of exercise.

THE HAZARDS OF FAD DIETS

Fad diets sound great. Just follow a few simple rules, and watch the weight melt away. The problem is, those rules often severely restrict certain kinds of foods and may have you eating abnormally large quantities of others. The infamous grapefruit diet, for example, has followers eating grapefruit to the virtual exclusion of all other foods. (The premise is that grapefruit "burns" fat, though no scientific evidence indicates this.) Certainly you will lose weight with such a diet—at first. Such diets do not provide nearly the level of calories your body needs for its daily functions, forcing it to convert glycogen (carbohydrates stored in your body's muscles and liver) and fat to produce energy. Many fad diets are nutritionally inadequate as well. Not only do they provide insufficient calories, but they also shortchange your body of needed nutrients found in the foods that are on the "no" list. Foods on the "yes" list (which is typically quite short) often are high in water content (such as grapefruit) or fiber (such as rice), giving you the sensation of eating something substantial that really is not.

Diets that severely restrict calories to fewer than 1,000 a day are often counterproductive. You might lose weight rapidly when you first begin such a diet, but your body quickly shifts into starvation mode and slows metabolism as a way to protect itself from such a drastic loss. This lowers the number of calories it needs, lessening the effect of the restricted intake. Much of the early weight loss is actually water, not fat. Such very low-calorie diets are unpleasant because you feel hungry and uncomfortable most of the time. Rebound weight gain is a particular problem once you stop the diet, as your body returns to more normal calorie needs.

Most fad diets are time-limited. The goal is to force your body to lose weight quickly. Once that goal is met, the diet has served its purpose and you return to your regular eating habits. More often than not, you return to your previous weight as well, because **you have not made the long-term changes in your lifestyle that will keep your weight at the appropriate level**. Many people also find that weeks of deprivation lead to irresistible cravings. They may reach their weight goals, then spend days indulging in all the foods they were not allowed to eat on the fad diet.

It is not always easy to identify a fad diet. Some are developed or sponsored by people who appear to be legitimate experts in health and nutrition. Some of these sponsors may believe they have actually stumbled across a true "cure" for obesity, and want to share the good news of their discovery with those who can benefit from it the most. However, most fad diets tend to benefit the bank accounts of those who come up with them, doing little for the health and well-being of the people who follow them. Most health professionals, from nutritionists and wellness experts to doctors, will recite the all-too-familiar refrain, "Eat fewer fats and carbohydrates, eat more fruits and vegetables, and exercise more." This is the tried and true formula that brings about weight loss in nearly everyone.

THE RISKS OF DIET PREPARATIONS AND DRUGS

Some people do not lose weight easily, despite their best efforts to follow the familiar formula. Those who are severely obese (a BMI of 30 or greater, or a BMI of 27 or greater if there are significant health problems present) may benefit from medical intervention such as medication or surgery (more about this later in this chapter). Those who want to lose more moderate amounts of weight are often tempted to boost their efforts with diet aids (available over the counter) or diet drugs (which require a prescription from a doctor).

If diet preparations or drugs are used in a medically supervised program of weight loss, **where you also learn healthy eating and exercise habits to make permanent changes in your lifestyle**, these substances can be helpful. The trouble is, this does not always happen. Especially with over-the-counter preparations, there is a tendency to rely on the product to handle the weight loss. But these substances are only aids. They are not magic pills that suck fat from your body while you sleep. You must still participate by learning new (and nutritious) eating habits and increasing your level of physical activity.

AVOID THE "YO-YO" SYNDROME

First you lose weight, and life is great. You buy an entire new wardrobe to celebrate. Six months later, nothing fits. The pounds are back, and they brought reinforcements. Welcome to the "yo-yo" syndrome, or weight cycling, the bane of every dieter. Weight cycling occurs because weight loss has focused on a short-term goal, typically to lose a certain amount of weight. People reduce calories and increase exercise until they meet their goals, and then return to their previous lifestyle habits. Because those habits allowed weight to become a problem in the first place, it is inevitable that without changing them, lost weight will return. The key to breaking this cycle is to make permanent changes in your eating and exercise habits. These must become your new lifestyle habits. Then they will help you keep your weight under control.

Losing weight is a constant struggle for me. What can make it easier?

Some people who struggle to lose weight have metabolic

or genetic factors that make weight control an ongoing battle. For many people, however, the true battle is one of conflicting expectations. Our modern society is very fast-paced. We are accustomed to getting where we want to go or having what we want to have quickly and without much effort. Multilane roads and synchronized traffic signals ensure we can drive to shopping malls and office complexes without interruptions. Interstate freeways whiz us from one city to another in minutes. Jet airplanes zoom us across the country in less time than it takes to play a good game of Monopoly. Fast-food restaurants promise meals in minutes. We have come to expect this as our standard of living. We are not very good at accepting things that take time.

Losing weight is one of those things. It takes time to lose weight, just as gaining weight takes time. But most people do not notice those extra pounds accumulating because they add up just cells at a time. Sorry to be the bearer of unwelcome news, but that is how those extra pounds go away, too. The most effective weight-loss plan for most people is to find a balance between calories in and calories out that lets them lose between half a pound and two pounds a week. Yes, at this rate it could take four to six months to lose that extra 20 pounds you just noticed when you stepped on the scale for your annual physical exam. It probably took you six months to a year to put it on. But this is a rate of weight loss based on reasonable expectations. It requires you to slowly change your eating and exercise habits, which is the best way to have new habits replace old ones. (Chapter 9 provides more information about nutrition and exercise and their roles in weight management and health.)

JOIN A REPUTABLE WEIGHT LOSS PROGRAM

Some people benefit from joining a weight-loss program. These typically offer a clear structure to guide you to your weight-loss goals. Some programs have strong educational components and emphasize learning the "whys" behind the diet and exercise recommendations. Others provide prepackaged foods and schedules for when and what to eat. Although this makes it easier to limit calories, it does not help you learn how to choose and prepare nutritious foods and appropriate servings for yourself. Programs that use liquid food replacements may not provide the nutritional elements your body needs, including fiber. Some weight-loss programs have a set price for a specific set of services. Others charge according to how much weight you lose or how many sessions you attend.

If you are considering a weight-loss program, try to talk with someone who has previously used the same one. It is best if the person has been out of the program for some time, so you can get a sense for how effective the methods have been in not just dropping pounds but also in keeping them off. Find out exactly what your money buys when you enroll, and what features are integral to the program but cost extra (such as prepackaged meals or support group meetings). Check to see what happens when the most intense portion of the program ends. Are there continuing support groups? Can you call the nutritionist if you have questions? Will you be able to continue weight loss or maintain your weight on your own, or does the program expect you to continue using its products (including prepackaged meals)? Also check with consumer advocacy groups in your area, too, such as the Better Business Bureau or the Chamber of Commerce, to see if there are complaints about the program.

CONSULT WITH A NUTRITIONIST OR DIETICIAN

Most hospitals and many larger medical centers have licensed nutritionists or dieticians who can help you develop nutritious menus and meal plans to lose weight safely and consistently. Some require a referral from your doctor so they understand the medical goals and any relevant health circumstances, such as diabetes or dyslipidemia, that could affect dietary recommendations. A nutritionist can help you develop a gradual substitution plan, replacing high-carbohydrate, high-fat foods with more nutritious but still tasty alternatives. We do not typically think about learning how to eat, which becomes a major stumbling block for many people trying to make changes in their eating habits.

ENROLL IN ACTIVITY CLASSES

Community centers and health clubs often offer a variety of activities ranging from aerobic dance to yoga, basketball to swimming. Being around other people who are having a good time working up a sweat is a great way to shift your mindset about exercise. When you join a class or a group, what was once work becomes fun. It is easier to make something a part of your daily routine when you enjoy it. And on those days when you just cannot muster any enthusiasm for exercise, knowing your classmates will want to know why you did not show up might be incentive enough to drag yourself to class even though you would rather go home and crash on the couch.

I have tried to lose weight, but always seem to gain back what I lost and then some. Now my weight is causing serious health problems. Will medication or surgery help?

Prescription medications or surgery may be weight-loss solutions for some individuals who are severely obese. These approaches are not for everyone who is obese, however, and lifestyle changes are still essential to maintain a healthy weight. If you have questions about weight-loss medications or surgeries, ask your doctor.

PRESCRIPTION MEDICATIONS
FOR WEIGHT LOSS

Most prescription medications used to assist with weight loss target chemicals in the brain that regulate appetite. Many of these drugs have potentially serious side effects, so they are prescribed for people whose BMI is greater than 30, or whose BMI is greater than 27, and who have serious medical conditions related to obesity. Prescription diet drugs are most effective when they are incorporated into a comprehensive program that also includes nutritional counseling, exercise guidance, and behavioral modification. Some of the newer drugs on the market target the body's digestive process, aiming to interfere with the absorption of fats. These do not have the same kinds of side effects as the medications that alter brain chemicals.

SURGERY FOR WEIGHT REDUCTION

Surgery is usually an intervention of last resort for people who are morbidly obese (generally more than 100 pounds overweight or who have a BMI of 40 or greater), who have been unable to lose weight through other means, and whose health is in jeopardy because of obesity-related diseases. The surgeries with the highest success rates are gastric stapling and gastric bypass, both of which reduce the stomach to a small pouch that can hold only an ounce or two of food. Sometimes the surgery also bypasses a section of the small intestine, reducing the body's ability to absorb nutrients as food passes through.

Surgery is not a quick fix, however. While most people do lose weight, few lose as much as they would like to lose. Most lose 40 to 50 percent, enough to drop them into a lower-risk BMI but not enough to get them to an ideal weight. Weight management after surgery requires commitment to lifestyle changes in eating habits and exercise. Without these changes, weight will gradually creep back up. Eating more food than the stomach's streamlined capacity causes nausea and vomiting. Some people who continue to eat more food than the stomach can hold end up stretching it back to near original size, defeating the intent of the surgery. Rapid weight loss also tends to cause loss of muscle as well, a problem until the body readjusts to its new size. There can also be complications from the surgery, since obesity interferes with healing. Recovery is really a lifelong process.

Will over-the-counter appetite suppressants help me feel less like eating?

Over-the-counter appetite suppressants often contain mild stimulants such as caffeine and various forms of ephedrine. They rely on the tendency of stimulants to make you feel less hungry and less like eating. The extent of this effect varies among those who take the preparations. Some people experience enough appetite suppression to avoid snacks and eat moderate amounts at meals. Other people can go most of the day without feeling the need to eat, then suddenly have an attack of the hungries during which they eat more than they would have had they snacked throughout the day. Many over-the-counter appetite suppressants produce unreliable effects within the individuals who take them as well. The product may work well for a few days, then not have any effect at all for a few days.

Most appetite suppressants also come with a recommended diet for you to follow while taking the product. Some of these recommendations are nutritious and safe, while others are variations on popular fad diets. A nutritious diet combined with regular exercise will result in weight loss without an appetite suppressant for most people.

Stimulants such as those in many over-the-counter appetite suppressants make your heart beat faster, your pulse accelerate, and your blood pressure rise. If you take more than the recommended dose, or take the product for longer than is recommended, you can experience a number of adverse reactions including heart palpitations (the sensation that your heart is fluttering), nervousness and anxiety, and difficulty sleeping. Your body may also develop an insensitivity to the product if you take it for a long time, which means you will have to take more of it to get the same effect. Be wary of herbal diet preparations as well. Many contain ephedra, a stimulant that becomes ephedrine in your body.

Some over-the-counter diet preparations attempt to interfere with digestion by preventing certain substances from being absorbed into your body. Some of these incorporate various forms of fiber. One is called chitosan, an indigestible starch found in the shells of shrimp and crab. As chitosan goes through your intestines, it binds with some of the fat, keeping it from being digested as well. This might not be such a bad thing except for one detail: It also binds with fat-soluble vitamins, keeping them from being absorbed into your body. It is best to check with your doctor before using such preparations, particularly if you are taking any medications.

If losing body fat is the issue, can I have liposuction and just get rid of the extra fat all at once?

It certainly is appealing to think you could just have extra fat sucked right out of your body and forget about the tedium of diet and exercise! If this were the case, there would certainly be far fewer overweight people, not to mention very long lines at the plastic surgeon's office. Though liposuction is the most commonly performed cosmetic surgery in the United States, it is not an efficient way to lose body fat. Most people who have liposuction are at most slightly overweight and want to remove small amounts of excess fat from specific areas.

Liposuction was first introduced in the early 1970s. Early liposuction procedures were painful and messy, causing bleeding that left much bruising and swelling. Newer techniques have significantly reduced these side effects, though they are not without risk. Recovery is still fairly long (at least a few weeks) and painful. Infection and reaction to the topical anesthetic drugs sometimes used can result in serious medical problems and even death. People who have cardio-vascular disease, peripheral vascular disease (poor circula-tion in the extremities), and diabetes are at particular risk for complications and are not usually considered appropriate patients for liposuction procedures.

Weight loss is not the primary objective of liposuction, and it is usually limited to less than 20 pounds with each procedure. Removing a greater volume than this or remov-ing smaller amounts of fat from multiple body areas increases the risk of complications. Liposuction perma-nently removes fat cells, leading many people to believe the fat loss is permanent. Your body cannot grow new fat cells, so you cannot regain fat in areas where the fat cells have been removed. But you can continue to gain weight in other parts of your body. Only nutritious eating habits and regular exercise can prevent this from happening.

Can I be overweight and healthy?

It is possible to be technically overweight and be very healthy, if you have a lot of lean body tissue and are physi-cally active. A good example is a professional athlete who has a lot of muscle mass. Muscle weighs more than fat, so on a chart an athlete might appear overweight. This is one reason many doctors prefer other measurement systems to assess whether a person is "overfat." It is body fat, not nec-essarily body weight, that poses potential health problems.

The BMI is not always a good measure of body fat in peo-ple who have a lot of lean body mass (toned and developed muscles). Other measures of body fat might be necessary to be sure you are not overfat. This includes measuring the fat between folds of skin on the back of your arm using special calipers, or a water displacement test.

I thought it was natural to gain a few pounds as you got older. Should I really weigh the same when I am 50 years old as I did when I was 20?

The "natural" tendency to gain weight as we grow older is partly what worries doctors. For many years, we did believe a certain amount of weight gain with age was a normal and acceptable aspect of growing older. We also believed it was "natural" to develop heart disease, arthritis, and other health problems. This was before we understood the relationship between being overweight and developing these conditions.

The old weight charts divided acceptable weight ranges into age categories. Current recommendations for healthy weight do not do this. There is strong evidence that a weight gain of 20 pounds or more during your early and middle adult years (from about age 20 to age 55) signals an increased risk for health problems. One long-term study of heart disease coincidentally found that most people will gain this amount during these years unless they modify their eating and exercise habits. Body metabolism appears to slow somewhat as we get older, and cell functions are not as efficient. Muscle tissue diminishes and fat tissue increases. This means the body needs less fuel. Most people continue eating at the same level they always have, however, which slowly becomes excessive. The body converts the excess to fat, further increasing the percentage of body fat. Researchers believe this is one factor contributing to the increased likelihood of insulin resistance in people over age 40 or so. Based on this new understanding of the relationship between aging and body fat, most health experts no longer believe weight gain is an inevitable aspect of aging. They recommend that people begin cutting back on the amount of food they eat and maintain regular physical activity as they enter their thirties, forties, and fifties to prevent age-related weight gain.

9

Taking Care of Yourself:
Nutrition and Exercise

Feasts have been a favorite form of celebration throughout history, honoring harvests, holidays, triumphs, and passages. Records that have survived from medieval England list the ingredients for a 165-pound Christmas pie measuring nine feet across: two bushels of flour, 20 pounds of butter, four geese, four ducks, two dozen assorted smaller birds, a pair of rabbits, and two cow tongues. Presumably this intriguing delicacy fed an entire village! Wealthy ancient Romans, noted for their culinary extravagance, threw lavish feasts that often lasted for days.

In these times, of course, feasting was more than social. There were few ways to preserve perishable food items. Unless foods were eaten, they rotted. Insects and rodents attacked stored grains, eating more than they left. This meant that food was plentiful through the summer and fall, and scant in the winter and spring. People ate as much as they could during times of abundance so they could survive during times of scarcity. Researchers believe people living in these early cultures were genetically programmed to do this, much as some animals are genetically programmed to hibernate. (See the discussion of the thrifty gene theory in Chapter 8.)

OUR CULTURE OF EXCESS

Many Americans eat far more food than their bodies
require. Nutritionists consider a serving of meat, for example, to be 3 ounces—about the size of a deck of cards. Yet
those steaks you throw on the grill may be 8, 10, 12, even 16
ounces or more—a full pound! Product packaging can be
particularly confusing, leading you to believe that the item
contained within is a single serving when in fact it is not. A
16-ounce bottle of soda might be labeled as containing two
servings, but you are probably going to drink all of it yourself.

Portion sizes have been on a steady increase since the
1950s, especially for food served in restaurants. "All you
can eat" restaurants draw large crowds. This pun is inten-
tional—people who eat regularly at such establishments typically weigh more than they should. This is in part because
they overeat and partly because the food is often high in fats
and carbohydrates. Often, a fast-food meal exceeds the *total*
daily recommended amounts of calories as well as fats and
carbohydrates, yet most fast-food restaurants will gladly
"up-size" your meal for a small additional charge.

Many health experts believe overeating leads to far more
significant problems than just weight gain. Large volumes of
food put a great strain on the body's resources, literally
stretching the capacity of the stomach and digestive system.
Most people who overeat do not splurge on broccoli and
bananas, either. It is those cookies and pastries, pastas and
potatoes, cheeseburgers and snack chips that sing the siren
song of temptation. These items are high in carbohydrates,
fats, or both. Researchers believe such foods contribute significantly to insulin resistance.

OUR SEDENTARY SOCIETY

What was your last physical activity? More than half of
all Americans get no more exercise than walking to and

from the refrigerator during television commercials. We have become a culture of couch potatoes. Many health experts believe this sedentary lifestyle is a direct path to an early grave. To stay healthy and fit, the human body must stay active. Activity generates energy, and energy keeps all these intricate systems in our bodies working smoothly and efficiently.

At the beginning of the twentieth century, discoveries that made work easier revolutionized the world. Machinery began to take over many physical tasks previously handled by people, and people shifted to operating the machinery. Over the next decades, continuing advances in technology further refined automation in nearly every aspect of life. No longer do people walk several miles to and from school or work, stand over a hot stove for hours a day to prepare meals, or even rake the autumn leaves from the yard. Cars, buses, and trains have nearly eliminated walking as a means of transportation. Microwave ovens can move a meal from the freezer to the table in just minutes. Power blowers whisk away lawn debris with no more effort than it takes to stand in the yard.

There are many benefits from all the automation that make our lives easier, safer, and more comfortable, of course. But we have overlooked the need to change our lives to keep them active. After viewing physical labor as something to be conquered for so long, it is a difficult transition to now see it as something that kept our bodies healthy and strong—and something we must replace to remain healthy and strong.

What is nutrition?

Diet and nutrition are two important aspects of weight management and of health in general. We tend to think of "diet" as something we do when we want to lose weight and "nutrition" as something related to substances in our food that we cannot see or taste. In reality, diet and nutrition are distinct but inseparable. Your diet is your pattern of eating—

what you eat, how much you eat, and when you eat. Nutrition is the act of nourishing your body through the foods you eat. Your diet supplies your body with the nutrients it needs to function. How well it does so depends on what, when, and how much you eat.

CARBOHYDRATES AND SUGARS

Carbohydrates are the source for most of your body's energy. Most health experts feel that simple, processed sugars are not healthy in large amounts. The more complex carbohydrates are better, in terms of the slowness of digestion and metabolism. The more fiber that is in carbohydrates also makes them better, and cause less rapid glucose rise. Current federal guidelines suggest that about half of a day's food intake should come from carbohydrates. Many doctors feel this is too high and recommend that carbohydrates make up about 35% to 40% of your daily calories. Cereal, grain, and fruit are common sources of carbohydrates, as are products made from them such as bread and pasta. Some diets that recommend that half of the calories come from carbohydrates are not designed for people who have the conditions of syndrome X. Doctors recommend a diet lower in carbohydrates for people with syndrome X.

PROTEINS

Proteins metabolize into amino acids, which are important for many functions at the cell level (especially cell growth and repair). Proteins are commonly found in animal products, including meat and dairy items. Proteins associated with the least animal (saturated) fats and cholesterol are preferred, and lean is healthier than fatty. Good sources of animal proteins include white-meat poultry (chicken and turkey), fish, and lean cuts of beef and pork. Fish that is high in omega-3 fatty acids may also have other specific advantages, particularly for heart health. Vegetable sources of protein include lentils, beans, and legumes. Vegetable proteins contain no cholesterol.

FATS

Most health experts recommend that only 20% to 30% of your daily food intake come from fatty foods. Your body needs some fat for cell activities. The typical American diet is nearly 40% fat, however. Not all fat is equal. Saturated fats (fats that are solid at room temperature, usually from animal sources) contribute to high blood cholesterol and other unhealthy lipid levels, which are major factors in heart disease. Poly- and monounsaturated fats (which take a liquid or semisolid form at room temperature) are from plant and fish sources and are considered healthier. Omega-3 fatty acids, found in certain fish, are believed by some to carry special protection against heart disease and cancer.

FIBER

Fiber is an important substance in digestion, helping to bind other food products so they can travel through the digestive system. Fiber also absorbs some cholesterol and may help to lower the glycemic index of certain foods. Fruits, vegetables, and whole grains are good sources of fiber.

VITAMINS AND MINERALS

Vitamins and minerals are necessary for metabolism. A nutritious, balanced diet provides the minerals and vitamins most people need. The federal government has established minimum daily recommended amounts for the most common vitamins and minerals. Women (and sometimes men) who do not consume dairy products may need additional calcium. Vitamin and mineral supplements are intended to augment a nutritious diet, not replace it. Though many people believe taking additional vitamins and minerals is beneficial, scientific evidence to support this is contradictory. Some substances can be harmful or fatal in large amounts, such as fat-soluble vitamins and minerals, including iron and zinc.

How do I translate good nutrition into a healthy diet?

This is an area of incredible controversy and many unanswered questions. There are very few absolute truths and many opinions. The federal government has attempted to address this issue to establish consistency in food-labeling practices as well as health recommendations. For several decades, a system known as the four basic food groups ruled nutritional guidelines. Foods were divided into the milk group, the meat group, the fruit-and-vegetable group, and the bread-and-cereal group. Recommendations included both serving size and number of servings. Then further research revealed more about the role of nutrients in the body and their sources, and nutritionists created the food pyramid, which reorganized and expanded the food groups. The number of recommended servings also changed. These guidelines frame many government nutrition programs, including school lunch programs and meal services for the elderly.

Most nutritionists find the food pyramid useful for demonstrating the varieties of foods that should make up your daily intake, but feel it is too general to be a valuable tool for meal planning. Many health experts also believe the food pyramid's recommendation for 50% of daily calories to come from carbohydrates is too high. These professionals suggest a diet that is lower in carbohydrates and higher in fruits and vegetables. This is often the recommendation for people who have insulin resistance, diabetes, and other syndrome X conditions that appear influenced by carbohydrates and glucose.

There is much debate in the medical community about the roles of simple and complex carbohydrates and how they affect insulin sensitivity and blood glucose levels. This has resulted in the concept of a glycemic index—a way of looking at foods according to how they are likely to affect blood insulin and glucose levels. Foods that digest quickly into sugars have a high glycemic index, while those that digest slowly have a low glycemic index. This system has become the basis for a number of diet plans. However, many doctors and nutritionists believe that a well-balanced, nutritious diet offsets the effects that high–and low–glycemic index foods might independently have on blood sugar and insulin levels. Any potential problem with wide fluctuations occurs when the diet is significantly higher in carbohydrates than other nutrients.

What are calories, and why do they matter?

A calorie is a unit of measure for energy. (Technically, it is the amount of energy it takes to raise the temperature of 1 gram of water 1 degree Celsius.) In nutritional terms, calories measure the energy equivalency of foods. Not all foods are equal when it comes to calories. One gram of fat has more than twice as many calories as 1 gram of protein or carbohydrate. This means that fat provides more energy for your body per gram—and your body must expend more energy to "burn" fat.

Most people, especially those trying to lose weight, focus on calories when planning meals. This can be helpful in getting a general sense of energy in and energy out. The average human body uses between 1,000 and 3,000 calories of energy a day, depending on your activity level. A diet that supplies this same level will maintain your present weight. A diet that supplies fewer calories will result in weight loss. However, there are other factors to consider. A diet that is low in calories is not necessarily nutritious, especially if many of those calories come from fat. (A high-calorie diet is not necessarily nutritious, either.)

Many doctors suggest keeping calorie counting as the background and focusing on eating a well-balanced, nutritious diet. This shifts the emphasis from weight loss to health improvement. If you are eating nutritiously, you are eating more fruits and vegetables that are as low in calories as they are high in nutrients. So you get the same result—lower calorie intake—but within a different framework. Though this may seem more like semantics than science, remember that what you are trying to do is change your lifestyle habits for the long term. Losing weight is just a short-term aspect of that goal. You are trying to reorient your perspective on food. This is most successful when you can look at food in terms of nutritional value in addition to calorie counting.

How do I know what nutrients are in the foods I am eating?

Packaged food products are labeled to identify their nutritional value and content, including fat and carbohydrate content, serving size, and number of calories. Such quantifications are obtained in laboratories where scientists measure and analyze every aspect of the product. Foods that come straight from nature are not so easily distilled to their base nutritional ingredients. The food pyramid provides some good general guidelines for selecting foods according to their nutritional value.

Assessing the nutritional value of foods becomes quite tricky when you are looking at a full meal, particularly in a restaurant. Start by identifying the core food items. Then identify what has been added to them, such as sauces or cheese. How was the food prepared? Fried foods generally have less nutritional value because they have added fat and because this method of cooking typically drains nutrients.

Broiled and baked foods usually have no added fats, though they could have sugars and other condiments that boost their fat and carbohydrate content. Canned foods may have little nutritional value.

READING FOOD PRODUCT LABELS

Federal regulations require packaged foods to display a label listing the item's nutritional information. All labels contain the same kind of information so you can easily compare one product to another. This can help you choose a can of tomato soup that is low in fat and sodium, for example. Food product labels also list the percentage of the daily recommended value a particular substance accounts for. This helps you determine whether you are exceeding a certain category, such as fat or carbohydrate.

Many restaurants have similar listings for their most common menu items. You usually have to request this information, and you may have to write to the restaurant's corporate office. This is worthwhile if you eat out frequently.

NATURAL AND ORGANIC FOODS

Many people believe foods that are organic (grown without chemicals) or natural (processed and packaged without additives or preservatives) provide more nutrition than other foods. This is not necessarily true. These terms, *natural* and *organic*, refer to how these products are grown or processed. For the most part, nutritionally a tomato is a tomato. What can matter is how fresh it is. Vegetables and fruits are highest in vitamins, minerals, and other nutrients when eaten right after harvesting. For this reason, vegetables you grow yourself might have more nutritional value than those you buy in the grocery store because you can pick them right before you eat them. Because natural and organic foods are chemical-free, many people believe they are healthier. This is difficult to measure scientifically, and has little to do with their nutritional value. However, because natural and organic foods do not contain additives and preservatives, they are often fresher. This can affect their nutritional value.

Packaged and processed foods lose some nutritional value as an aspect of processing. Organic frozen green beans have less vitamins and minerals than organic fresh green beans because the process of freezing them removes some nutrients. The same thing happens with commercially grown green beans—and other vegetables and fruits. Canning draws the most nutrients from foods. Canned green beans may contain less than 10% of the nutrients they had when first picked. Cooking them destroys even more, partly as a result of heating them and partly to nutrients that leach into the water usually added during cooking. Many nutritionists believe canned vegetables and fruits have virtually no nutritional value by the time they reach the table.

The best way to get maximum nutritional value from the foods you eat is to eat them in forms that are close to those found in nature. Whole apples and oranges have more nutritional value than juices made from the fruits. So do whole grain breads. Whenever possible, buy fresh produce and eat it raw, or cook it as little as possible. This matters more, from a nutritional perspective, than whether the items are organically grown.

How much should I eat?

A general rule of thumb is that if you are maintaining your ideal weight, you are eating the right amount. If you are gaining weight, you are eating too much (and probably exercising too little). If you are losing weight without intending to, you might be eating too little or have other health concerns your doctor should evaluate.

There are different ways to look at how much you eat. The

federal government issues guidelines that suggest average daily calories, and this is how many people are used to measuring food. The food pyramid, also government issue, suggests daily serving quantities and sizes. Packaged foods such as bread, canned goods, condiments, and other items are labeled to identify what quantity is considered a single serving. This can be confusing when the labeled serving size differs from the way the product is typically eaten. Most bread, for example, identifies one slice as a serving. Making a sandwich with two slices of bread, then, constitutes two servings. Before looking at how much you *should* eat, you need to first look at how much you *do* eat.

Many people underestimate how much they eat, partly because they misinterpret serving sizes and partly because they consume items without thinking of them as foods. A can of peas might be labeled as containing three servings, though you might be accustomed to eating the entire can as a single serving. That swipe of mayonnaise on each slice of your sandwich bread is probably two servings, too (with a typical serving size of 1 tablespoon). That morning latte that jolts you awake could have as many as 600 calories, depending on how you order it, as well as half your day's allotment of fat. Even a simple cup of coffee can contain 100 or more hidden calories if you add sugar and cream. (And beware that nonfat, nondairy substitute, which is more than likely all sugar.)

How you serve your food makes a difference in how much you eat as well. The appropriate serving of canned peas, for example—one-third can—looks pretty small in a bowl. Yet it fills an appreciable space on a plate. A sandwich made with one slice of bread (a half-sandwich) may appear lonely on a dinner plate, yet fills a luncheon or salad plate. If you are accustomed to eating by your eyes, proper serving sizes will look too small. The key is to retrain your eyes by presenting food differently. Use smaller dishes to make portions appear larger. Measure servings, if necessary, to be

sure you have the correct amount. It will take some time, but
eventually your eyes will adjust to seeing these amounts as
adequate and even filling.

When I try to cut back on eating, I feel hungry all the time. How can I avoid this?

In some respects, the key concept is "feel." The actual
sensation of hunger results from a complex series of reactions. When blood sugar levels drop, cells do not receive the
fuel they need to function properly. They complain to a
grape-sized area in the brain, the hypothalamus. The hypothalamus signals the stomach to get busy, and the stomach
responds by releasing acid to initiate the digestive process.
But digestion cannot go far without food, which is your
responsibility. The release of acid causes the stomach to
churn and gurgle, producing an unpleasant and almost
painful sensation.

While all of us experience the sensations of hunger when
it has been several hours since our last meal, such as first
thing in the morning, many people believe they feel hungry
when they know it is time to eat. This is really your appetite
at work, not hunger. Your appetite is what tells you to eat
things that smell, look, and taste good—sometimes when
you actually are hungry, and sometimes when you are not
hungry but encounter the sights and smells of foods. Your
appetite is also to blame when you keep on eating even after
your stomach is satisfied.

People sometimes talk about their stomachs "shrinking"
when they diet. This is not quite what happens. A typical
"diet" reduces the amount of food you eat to reduce the calories you take in. After a few days to a week of reduced food
intake, your mind learns there will be no more food and
stops pestering you to eat more. As long as you are eating
enough to meet your body's calorie needs, your appetite
becomes more synchronized with your stomach's signals—
when your stomach is full, your appetite backs off.

Some diets so severely restrict calorie intake, however,

that your body does not get enough nutrients. Your body then goes into starvation mode, slowing metabolism to use less energy and thus need less fuel (food). This is an automatic, life-preserving process. Your cells do not know you are doing this to them intentionally—they only know that suddenly they do not have enough fuel to function. Though you may initially experience rapid weight loss with such a diet, you may also feel tired and low on energy. You are highly likely to regain the lost weight (and even more) when you return to less restrictive eating habits because your "starved" cells will rev up their metabolism in an attempt to restore your body to its previous condition (which had become normal).

Some people cut back too much without realizing it, or without recognizing the consequences. Some people make food choices that are not very satisfying. If you really do not like carrots, do not feel compelled to eat them. There are many other foods that can provide the same nutrients. Yet many people who are trying to lose weight feel they have to eat certain foods and give up others. Remember that you are trying to change your eating habits for life, not just to lose a few pounds. Moderation is more likely to make this successful. Feel free to experiment with different foods, to see which ones leave you feeling satisfied and which ones leave you longing for more. Look at this as a process not of giving up your favorite foods, but rather as a process of developing new favorites. Choose healthy, low-fat snacks to give you energy between meals.

How do I change my eating habits to lose weight or maintain a healthy weight?

The best way to change your eating habits is slowly but steadily, so the changes become your regular habits.

Changing your eating habits alone is not enough, however. At the same time, it is essential to increase physical activity. This raises cell metabolism, keeping the body's cells active enough to burn more, not less, energy. The value of this approach is twofold. First, it keeps your cells from going into starvation mode. This assures a steady supply of nutrients, and you feel more invigorated. Second, it bumps up your "metabolic thermostat." They start running higher and hotter, so to speak, and over time this becomes the new norm.

That nasty *w* word sometimes comes up—*willpower*. It does take determination and commitment to make any sort of a change; there is no way around that. Your eating habits are no exception. Sometimes you have to force yourself to do the right thing, to find ways to distract yourself from the foods that seem to be calling you. Occasionally your willpower will slip. This is normal. It does not mean you are a bad person. No one does everything exactly right all the time. Just move on. You cannot change what has already happened—you cannot retrieve that candy bar once you have eaten it. Let it go. It is not a failure, or even a setback. It was just a choice you made. Just do not follow it with four more candy bars. Make your next snack or meal a nutritious one. If you really feel that you have to "punish" yourself, take a walk. You will feel better in many ways, guaranteed.

TIPS FOR MORE NUTRITIOUS EATING

- **Eat less, but do not deprive yourself**. Most people who are overweight do need to reduce the amount of food they eat. Many restrictive diets severely reduce or even eliminate certain kinds of foods, depriving your body of needed nutrients. A far more effective approach is to reduce portion sizes so you still eat a variety of foods, just less of them.

- **Eat more foods that are nutritiously sound, and fewer foods that are nutritionally empty**. Many people also need to change the kinds of foods they eat, from those that are high in fat and sugar to those that are not. If you eat a lot of pastries and sweets, gradually transition to fruits that can satisfy your sweet tooth with fewer calories, less fat, and more nutritional value.

- **Avoid eating alone**. Most of us are more aware of what we eat when there are others around, making more health-conscious choices. In a restaurant, we tend to order the broiled chicken instead of a bacon cheeseburger, or a salad with the house vinaigrette instead of blue cheese dressing. We tend to forego second (and third) helpings at home meals. Dining with others turns meals into social experiences. Talking with other people while you are eating encourages you to eat more slowly, to eat less, and to focus your attention on something besides eating. Of course, you cannot eat with others all the time. When you must eat alone, set a place for yourself at the table and serve your plate just as you would if others were joining you. Do not watch television or read while you eat. You are more likely to eat too fast and too much when your attention is too tightly focused somewhere else. If you are eating alone in a restaurant, choose a table near the door or close to other diners. This gives you the sense that you are not by yourself.

- **Make changes one at a time**. Once you make the decision to improve your health by gaining control over your weight, you naturally want to rush right into your new habits so you can soon see the results of your efforts. This is almost a form of self-sabotage. It is human nature to simultaneously resist change and expect instant results. Even your taste buds need time to get used to new flavors and textures. Make changes one at a time, and give them about two weeks to settle in before adding another. If you do not like something after a fair trial, give it up and try something different.

- **Concentrate on developing new favorites**. One problem with many weight-loss plans is that they seem to focus on what you cannot have. Your real mission should be to develop new favorites that you can eventually like better than your old favorites. This is not a process of depriving yourself, but rather of expanding your tastes and your interests. You may find that those old favorites lose their appeal after six months or so.

THE PSYCHOLOGY OF (OVER) EATING

We eat for many reasons, few of which have anything to do with hunger or nutrition in modern society. We eat to celebrate, to mourn, to socialize, to comfort ourselves—and sometimes for reasons we cannot explain. Some people who overeat as adults grew up in families where food was scarce, or was used to reward and punish. Some people use food as a control mechanism, either through overeating or undereating. When there are psychological and emotional issues underlying eating habits, it is often difficult to change the habits without first addressing the issues.

My job requires me to travel a lot. How do I eat nutritiously when I am on the road?

Many people who travel extensively have learned how to avoid the hazards and pitfalls of eating away from home. It is usually not practical to carry food with you, especially if you are traveling long distances or will be on the road for more than a couple of days. Many states also prohibit the transport of fresh fruits and vegetables across their borders, as a means of controlling food crop pests that might be hitching a ride. Here are some tips for nutritious travel.

- **Make arrangements for vegetarian meals on flights that serve food**. More than a few regular travelers believe the phrase "airline food" is a contradiction in terms. Many airlines have cut way back on what refreshments they serve to passengers, and often just pass out snacks. Some short commuter flights may offer just coffee, or nothing at all. Longer cross-country and international flights do typically offer a meal. Most airlines offer you the opportunity to order a special meal to accommodate dietary restrictions or preferences. Ordering vegetarian is a good way to avoid the "mystery meat" and other processed foods that typically go into an airline meal. Vegetarian meals usually come with fresh fruit and vegetables, a welcome treat when you travel.

- **Buy a few groceries at the store and fix yourself some simple but nutritious snacks**. Many motels and hotels offer rooms with microwave ovens and small refrigerators for little or no extra charge. The concierge or desk clerk can tell you if there is a grocery store nearby and can often arrange for someone to do some shopping for you (this part will usually cost extra). Some grocery stores also provide a delivery service. This can be less expensive than ordering room service and more convenient than going to the motel's restaurant, and also give you a wider selection of foods.

- **Choose restaurants that feature "heart healthy" or low-fat menu items**. Most traditional restaurants (where you sit down and someone serves you) offer menu items that are low in fats and carbohydrates. You can sometimes ask how a dish is prepared and request substitutions for high-fat or high-sugar ingredients. Most restaurants (even diners and cafés) will use an egg substitute instead of eggs in an omelet, for example, or serve low-fat milk instead of whole milk or cream with oatmeal and coffee.

- **Order à la carte or single food items.** Many hotel restaurants will let you order single-food items rather than a combination meal. You can often order a grilled chicken breast and steamed vegetables, for example. If you see the ingredients for what you would eat as a healthy meal at home in entrées listed on the menu, you can often mix and match individual items to create a similarly healthy meal on the road.

Beware the trap of traveling on an expense account. It is easy to eat more food and order more extravagant meals when someone else is picking up the tab. This "treat" can quickly add up to excess pounds.

I am already on a strict diet to help control my type 2 diabetes. Isn't that enough?

The diet recommended for people with diabetes is generally nutritious and healthy. If you are maintaining your weight and are getting at least 30 minutes of moderate physical exercise four or five days a week, then you are probably doing all the right things to keep yourself healthy. If your doctor has suggested a weight-reduction diet and this is what you are following, be sure to follow up with your doctor or nutritionist when you reach your ideal weight. You may need to make some adjustments as you shift from weight loss to weight maintenance. A diet plan to help you lose weight generally contains about 500 fewer calories each day than a diet plan for maintaining your ideal weight. And again, regular exercise is a critical component of any plan.

Do I have to give up sugar if I have diabetes?

Doctors once believed that because too much sugar in the blood caused problems in diabetes, that sugar should be severely restricted in the diet to reduce the amount of it that got into the blood. We now know considerably more about how the body metabolizes various foods into forms of sugar, and that dietary sugar is not necessarily your body's primary source of glucose. We also understand better the role of insulin and its relationship to blood sugar levels. Most people with diabetes can eat sugary foods on occasion, as long as their diabetes is well controlled and they include dietary sugar as part of their total carbohydrate intake. For those whose diabetes is not well controlled, dietary sugar can spike blood sugar levels because it does get into the bloodstream much faster than more complex carbohydrates that must first be digested and metabolized.

High amounts of dietary sugar really are not healthy for anyone. Excess sugar—whether from sugary foods or other carbohydrates and fats—represents nutritionally empty calories for your body. It will simply process and store them as fatty tissue.

What about sugar and fat substitutes?

Many sugar substitutes, such as those found in sugar-free candy, are more like "sugar light." Usually identified on the label as sugar alcohols, these substances generally have half to two-thirds of the calories in an equivalent amount of sugar. Mannitol and sorbitol are common sugar alcohols found in products marketed as sugar-free. Though technically this designation is correct, such products still contain carbohydrates and can affect your blood sugar levels. Sugar substitutes such as aspartame (Equal is one brand name) truly are sugar-free. They do not contain calories, so using them in moderation as sweeteners is fine. Be sure to read the list of ingredients for other substances that may contain carbohydrates or fats.

Many fat substitutes are also carbohydrates, making up for the texture and flavor of fat by adding sweetness. Common fat substitutes that are carbohydrates include dextrin, maltodextrin, cellulose, modified food starch, and almost any ingredient that is a "gum." And of course, these ingredients all add calories to the product, though usually (but not always) fewer than fat would add. Other fat substitutes, such as the NutraSweet product Simplesse, are made from proteins found in milk, egg whites, and whey. And some fat substitutes are actually fats that are chemically modified to make them harder for your body to digest. Olestra is the most commonly known of these. While Olestra acts and tastes like fat, its molecular structure prevents it from being absorbed into your body. In some people, this can cause digestive-system problems such as cramping and diarrhea.

Are there certain foods that are harmful for those who have syndrome X?

Saturated fats found in animal products such as milk and red meat increase your risk for atherosclerosis and other cardiovascular diseases. Some health experts believe high levels of simple carbohydrates, such as those found in processed foods, contribute to insulin resistance and high blood glucose levels.

Are there certain foods that are therapeutic for those who have syndrome X?

You cannot go wrong with fresh, raw fruits and vegetables, which are high in vitamins and minerals as well as antioxidants believed to be useful in preventing and combating disease. Fish that are high in omega-3 fatty acids, such as salmon and mackerel, might provide extra help with lowering blood lipids, especially triglycerides.

I don't really have time to exercise. Is exercise that important?

Exercise is critically important. Many health experts believe exercise and nutritious eating are two halves of a whole. One without the other is significantly less effective in weight control as well as maintaining optimal health.

Most of us lead very busy lives as we juggle the often competing needs and demands of work and family. It seems that we hit the floor running in the morning when the alarm clock rings and do not stop until we collapse in bed again fourteen or sixteen hours later. Even the most hectic schedules have a few minutes here and there for some physical activity, though. Use every opportunity to walk, even if just down the hall to talk with a coworker. Stand up and move around while you are on the telephone. Fidget. Anything that gets your body moving is activity, and activity uses energy.

As challenging as it might be, try your hardest to make time for more intense exercise. The ideal for heart health is to get 30 to 45 minutes of aerobic exercise three or four days a week. Activities that have high aerobic potential include jogging, bicycling (10 to 12 miles per hour, not a leisurely ride around the block), swimming, cross-country skiing, tennis, handball, racquetball, squash, volleyball, basketball, soccer, and ice or roller (also in-line) skating. Activities that have more moderate, yet still useful, aerobic potential include brisk walking, bowling, golf (if you walk the course, not ride in a cart), and downhill skiing.

What kinds of exercise are most effective?

The kinds of exercise that are most effective for you are the ones you enjoy. If you like doing something, the odds are high that you will continue doing it. If exercise is a chore, you will soon find ways to avoid it. *What* you do is far less important than that you do *something* that is physical.

- **The power of walking**. Walking can burn about five to seven calories a minute, depending on how much you weigh and how fast you walk. Walking is the easiest, most natural way to improve fitness. It is good for your sense of well-being, for muscle tone, and even for your bone strength. Best of all, walking requires no special equipment.
- **Go aerobic for your heart**. Activities that get your heart pumping and your blood flowing are good for your heart, lungs, and circulatory system. Swimming, jogging, bicycling, or even fast walking (all at

a moderate pace) three to five times a week for 30 to 60 minutes at a time are among the aerobic exercises that can do this. Aerobic activity also appears to be able to directly lower blood glucose levels. Aerobic exercise is good for your figurative heart, too—your feelings and emotions. Whether a brisk walk or an all-out run around the track, physical activity reduces stress.

- **Involve others**. Make regular physical activity a family event. Take daily walks together, and explore activities you all like on the weekends. If you live alone or your family refuses to join you, join other group activities through a community center or health club. You are more likely to stay involved in an activity if other people are expecting you to participate.

- **When time is short**. No matter what you do for a living, make your day as active as possible. Walk, take the stairs, pace while you are on the telephone or in meetings, stand and stretch. Just keep moving. These little efforts add up to big returns.

My weight goes up and down from day to day, and even during the day. How do I know how much I really weigh?

It is normal for your weight to fluctuate throughout the day, and from day to day, for reasons that have nothing to do with weight loss or gain. Despite its solid appearance, your body is mostly water. How much water your body contains at any given time depends on how much you have been eating and drinking, sweating, and urinating. It also depends on what you are doing, whether you are awake or asleep, sitting at a desk, or loading trucks. Women often notice hormonal weight changes, too, as their bodies retain fluid just before menstruation (yet another aspect of your body's preparation for a potential pregnancy). These weight fluctuations can be mere ounces that your scale barely detects or several pounds.

Get off the scale! These normal fluctuations will drive you nuts and are likely to undermine your efforts. Weigh yourself just once a week, on the same day and at the same time. Then forget about your weight until the next week. Concentrate instead on what else is happening to your body as you steadily improve your eating habits and increase your physical activity level. Your cells are working more efficiently. Your arteries are clearing. Your lungs can pull in more oxygen with each breath. Though these changes happen cell by cell and you may not see these results for a while, you can visualize them. This is a great way to shift your focus from your short-term goal of weight loss to your long-term goal of better health. You will eventually notice changes in your body as you make progress in changing your behaviors, even if you throw away your scale. Your clothes will loosen and your appearance will change. You will feel more energized and happier with yourself.

Remember that muscle weighs more than fat. It is common to get a few weeks or so into your new health and fitness plan, then see the scale creep up a bit. If other signs of weight loss are present—such as loosening clothes and more energy—you are most likely seeing the effects of increasing muscle mass as you are decreasing fat tissue. Do not panic—this will eventually even out as your body gets used to the new and improved you. Other factors to consider besides weight are your BMI and your waist measurement. If these are both edging downward, you are doing the right things. If you are following a nutritious diet and are exercising regularly, yet your weight keeps going up, contact your doctor. Occasionally, insulin-sensitizing medications do cause weight gain.

My weight is normal. Does that mean my eating habits are healthy?

You may well have healthy eating habits if your weight is normal. Other factors may also be saving you from the inevitable. Some people, especially younger men who are very active, seem able to eat just about anything without gaining weight. Their dietary excesses are still having an effect on their bodies, even if this is not obvious. Too much high-fat food can cause blood lipid levels to rise, which contributes to fatty buildup in the walls of the arteries. It is also possible to have too much body fat and still be within a normal weight range. It may also be that you are overweight (have too much body fat) but are in better physical condition overall because of regular exercise and more nutritious eating habits than someone who is of normal weight but does not eat properly or exercise regularly. Weight is not always a good measure of body fat or of health.

I think I need professional help to make all these changes. How do I find the right person or program?

Americans spend more than $30 billion a year on weight-loss products and programs. Many of these are at best useless and at worst can cause serious health problems. As clichéd as it is, if something sounds too good to be true, it is. The only known method to lose weight is to eat less and become more physically active. There are no creams, salves, body wraps, bracelets, magnets, pills, fad diets, concoctions, machines, gadgets, or gizmos that can take weight off for you. Gimmicks are plentiful, but all they will help you lose is your money. Losing weight and maintaining a healthy weight not only takes time but is a lifelong process.

People who are extremely obese (with a BMI of 40 or greater) should consult with a physician, often an internist or endocrinologist, who specializes in weight management. Your regular family doctor can usually refer you to someone reputable. If you live in a rural area, you may have to go to a large medical center to find such a specialist. Though this might seem like an inconvenience, consider it to be no different than traveling to see a specialist for cancer or heart disease. Obesity, especially extreme obesity, is no less serious a medical condition.

You should expect this specialist to do a comprehensive

physical exam that includes blood tests and a complete medical history. Many such specialists practice in weight-management clinics where they have immediate access to the resources of nutritionists, psychologists, exercise physiologists, and other health professionals. You may see some or all of these, depending on the specialist's assessment of your physical health and any underlying emotional issues.

Some people do well in consumer weight-loss programs that have strong education and support components. When considering such a program, be sure it focuses on developing more healthy habits, not just on weight loss. There should be classes in how to buy and prepare healthy foods, eat healthy in restaurants, resist cravings, and modify eating behaviors. There should also be a process for addressing potential underlying psychological issues (such as recommending a mental health therapist or psychologist who specializes in eating problems). No weight-loss program or diet plan can lose weight and improve health for you. It can only help you define and work toward your goals.

10

~

Looking Ahead to a
Bright (and Healthy) Future

Prevention and treatment efforts for the future are likely to be rooted at each end of the technology spectrum. For most people, particularly those who are at risk for syndrome X conditions but do not yet have them, prevention through healthy lifestyle habits remains a key focus. The more researchers learn about how nutrition and exercise affect the intricate functionings of the human body, the more we understand how much we can influence (and even control) through interventions as simple as changing what and how we eat. There is great hope that today's children may learn preventive and healthful eating habits while they are young, so they grow up to be adults with these habits already firmly entrenched. After all, changing lifestyle habits may be simple, but it is anything but easy to accomplish.

As researchers identify more genetic links for obesity and insulin resistance, they are gaining more insights into the roles these conditions play in health and wellness as well as in illness and disease. This understanding may well unlock the secrets of human survival through centuries of change. It could also fundamentally change the way we view health and illness, as we gain further understanding of the interactions between genetics, environment, and behavior. At this point in time, it does not appear that genetics alone establishes a condition within the syndrome X constellation, but rather it lays the foundation for a predisposition that is then influenced by environment and behavior. Whether future research will continue to support this hypothesis remains to be seen.

What complications are possible with the conditions of syndrome X, and how can I avoid them?

The complications of syndrome X conditions can be quite serious and are often compounded by the presence of more than one condition. For example, kidney disease is a potential complication of either diabetes or hypertension. When a person has both conditions, the risk for kidney disease rises substantially. Similarly, heart attack and stroke are potential complications of hypertension and dyslipidemia. Having both conditions compounds the risk for either complication. Other complications are unique to a particular condition. Infertility is a unique yet common complication of PCOS, for example, just as eye damage and blindness are complications of diabetes.

Fortunately, keeping your health conditions under good control and receiving regular medical care to discover developing complications before they become serious can prevent many situations from becoming serious. It is important to understand what complications are possible, how serious they can become, and what early signs and symptoms can alert you to them. Prevention and early intervention are the most effective approaches to reducing your risk for complications so you can enjoy a full and active life.

ADVANCED HEART DISEASE

Heart disease is the leading cause of death in the United States and is the most serious complication for most people with syndrome X conditions. Each condition contributes to and compounds the risk for developing advanced heart disease. Further, the risk increases exponentially. Having both hypertension and dyslipidemia, for example, does not just double your risk, it increases it six- or sevenfold. Keeping these conditions under control greatly reduces the risk, which is why early and appropriate treatment is so crucial.

Obesity places increased stress on the heart and circulatory systems. Fat tissue has a rich supply of blood vessels that add to the already extensive network of arteries, veins, and capillaries that make up the circulatory system. Mostly these vessels are capillaries, the smallest of the blood vessels. It takes considerable pressure to move blood to and through them. Getting blood to the capillaries is very important, since these are the conduits where the nutrient/waste exchange takes place. The red blood cells pass on oxygen and other nutrients, and pick up carbon dioxide and other wastes. The heart must beat harder and sometimes faster to push blood through all the extra tissues, which can lead to both cardiovascular disease and heart failure.

Other changes in the body that occur with obesity also affect the heart and blood vessels. Obesity, of course, is a condition not just of overweight but also overfat. Much of the extra fat has nowhere to go, and ends up lining the walls of the arteries. When this affects the arteries throughout the body, it causes arteriosclerosis and atherosclerosis. When it affects the arteries that supply the heart itself, it causes coronary artery disease. When the coronary arteries become occluded (plugged), surgery to unplug or bypass them is often the only recourse. Coronary artery bypass surgery is currently the most frequently performed operation in the United States.

Heart failure, generally the result of the heart muscle working too hard for too long, is more difficult to treat. There are many medications now available that slow the heart and reduce the force of each beat, helping to stem the damage. However, much heart failure is ultimately progressive, and results in exactly what the name implies—failure of the heart to adequately supply the body with blood. Once medications are no longer effective, the only solution is heart transplant. Not everyone with heart failure is a good candidate for transplant, however. The presence of other serious medical problems makes it highly unlikely that a transplant would be successful.

If you are being treated for any of the conditions of syndrome X, your doctor is probably monitoring you closely for any signs of developing heart disease. People with hypertension, diabetes, or dyslipidemia are at the greatest risk, since these conditions are considered tremendous risks for early forms of heart disease. Signs and symptoms that might indicate heart disease is developing include swelling of your feet and legs, shortness of breath in situations where breathing was not previously a problem, lightheadedness, and tightness in your chest. If you have any of these, have your doctor evaluate your condition.

Signs and symptoms of a heart attack include pain in your chest or radiating down your left shoulder and arm, difficulty breathing, a feeling of intense or crushing pressure in your chest, nausea, clamminess, and a feeling of very bad indigestion that does not go away after 15 minutes or so. **These signs can signal a life-threatening situation—see a doctor or go to a hospital emergency room immediately if you experience them**. While about two-thirds of those who have heart attacks survive, many of those in the third who do not survive might have done so if they had gone for immediate medical attention.

KIDNEY DISEASE

Between them, diabetes and hypertension account for nearly 60% of all end-stage renal disease in the United States. This is the final phase of kidney disease in which survival requires regular dialysis (using a machine to filter toxins from the blood) and kidney transplant. Nearly a quarter of a million Americans have end-stage renal disease. As many die from it as are newly diagnosed each year.

The kidneys are a pair of organs most people do not think much about until something goes wrong. Each about the size of a closed fist, they rest against your spine in the center of your back, just under your back ribs. About 50 gallons of blood flow through the intricate filtration system of your kidneys each day, which removes excess fluid and waste products. You pass about half a gallon of this as urine. Your kidneys also produce hormones and enzymes, play a role in producing red blood cells, and convert vitamins into other substances your body needs.

It is possible to live with one healthy kidney and experience no adverse effects. It is also possible to live with damaged kidneys for a very long time. In fact, there are few signs of kidney disease until the damage becomes extensive and they begin to fail. Early signs of kidney disease might include blood in the urine and swelling in your hands and feet or unexplained weight gain (signs of fluid retention). High blood pressure is another clue that kidney disease could be present, since kidney disease can also cause hypertension. Unfortunately, early signs are often vague and minor. It is not uncommon for a person to be unaware of kidney problems until kidney failure requires dialysis. Certain urine tests can help screen for indications that kidney function is not normal, and should be part of your regular medical care if you have hypertension or diabetes.

It appears that kidney functions can begin to change within the first five years or so after diabetes develops. These changes do not necessarily result in kidney disease, though about 20% to 40% of people who have diabetes do eventually develop it. The longer you have diabetes, the greater your risk. The risk is also higher for people with type 1 diabetes, though it is not clear whether this is related to a different disease mechanism or because type 1 diabetes typically starts early in life. And the risk is highest for people who have diabetes *and* hypertension. When kidney disease is detected early, there are a number of medical treatments that can slow the damage. Once it progresses to failure (the kidneys are unable to filter toxins and fluid from the blood), the only treatment is dialysis or transplant.

DIABETIC RETINOPATHY

Nearly 40,000 people a year lose their sight to diabetes. Diabetes causes changes in the blood vessels throughout the body. Those most severely affected are the tiniest, the capillaries. Within the eye, diabetes can cause new capillaries to grow across the retina, which is the light-sensitive "screen" onto which the cornea and lens of your eye project the images your brain interprets as vision. These diabetes-induced blood vessels are very fragile and rupture easily. When they rupture, the bleeding destroys sensitive nerves in the retinal tissue. The result is permanent damage that, if substantial, becomes blindness.

As with other potential complications, early diagnosis and intervention is essential—and early signs and symptoms are scant. Signs of early diabetic retinopathy, often called nonproliferative, or background, retinopathy, may include blurred vision and difficulty seeing close up. It is often hard to distinguish these changes from the normal changes that take place with advancing age. Most people over the age of 40 are beginning to experience the early stages of presbyopia, a natural loss of the eye's ability to focus on near objects. Sometimes, but not always, vision gets better and worse throughout the day. "Floaters," tiny bits of tissue that float around in the vitreous humor (the gelatinous fluid that fills the eyeball), are sometimes a sign of minor retinal bleeding, but again not always, and floaters are fairly common without relationship to eye disorders. Retinopathy that progresses to the stage where bleeding blood vessels cause permanent damage is called proliferative retinopathy. In this stage, the scar tissue that forms as a result of the bleeding can cause the retina to pull away from the back of the eye. This is called retinal detachment, and if not immediately repaired, can result in permanent blindness.

Laser surgery can often halt the progress of diabetic retinopathy, particularly if the disorder is detected and followed closely in the nonproliferative stage. If there has been a lot of bleeding into the vitreous, a procedure called a vitrectomy might be necessary. In this procedure, the eye surgeon removes the bloody vitreous and replaces it with a saline solution. This often restores clear vision.

INFERTILITY

About 40% of women who have PCOS also struggle with infertility. PCOS accounts for nearly half of infertility problems that are related to ovulation. The repeated formation and resorption of multiple ovarian cysts typically prevents ripe ova from being released, and also often scars the ovaries. Women with mild PCOS may not know they have the syndrome until they seek treatment for infertility, which then uncovers the underlying cause. Treatment with ovulation-stimulating drugs is often successful in women whose infertility is due to PCOS.

Are complications inevitable?

No. If the conditions of syndrome X are well controlled, there is no reason to expect that complications will develop. The risk always exists, of course. If the conditions of syndrome X are not well controlled, complications are more likely. It is especially important to understand the potential complications of the syndrome X conditions you have so you can take appropriate preventive actions as well as identify early symptoms.

How do I prevent more damage from occurring?

The most effective way to prevent further damage from occurring is to eliminate the risks that can be eliminated. Take any medications your doctor has prescribed for your medical conditions, and get regular checkups. Eat nutritiously and exercise regularly. While you may not be able to prevent all future health problems, you can often delay them.

How can I undo damage that has already occurred?

It depends on the damage. Unfortunately, not all damage can be undone, though some can be repaired. Coronary artery bypass surgery can restore the blood supply to the heart, for example, and a kidney transplant can replace damaged and nonfunctioning kidneys. But some health consequences are permanent. A stroke may leave residual paralysis, and proliferative retinopathy can cause irreversible blindness. Prevention really is the best approach. The earlier you start, the better—though it is never too late to make changes for a healthier lifestyle.

Will I have to take medications to treat my syndrome X conditions for the rest of my life?

In some people, lifestyle intervention can control and even reverse the features of conditions such as hypertension and type 2 diabetes. Other people will require medication to help them keep their symptoms under control in addition to lifestyle changes. There is no way to predict how your body will respond to treatment.

If I feel better and all of my levels (blood pressure, lipids, blood sugar) are normal, why do I still have to take medication?

Your levels are normal *because* you are taking medication. Though your signs have disappeared, you still have the condition that caused them. If you stop taking prescribed medication, it is very likely that your abnormal signs will return and may well be more severe. It can be very dangerous to suddenly stop taking some medications, especially those prescribed for high blood pressure. Successful treatment is not necessarily a cure, even though you may feel healthier than you ever have. Please, do not stop taking, or change the way you are taking, prescribed medications without first talking with your doctor.

What can I do to help my body heal itself?

At the risk of being repetitive, we have to say again—lifestyle. The best thing you can do for your body is to feed it nutritiously and exercise it regularly. Though this is not always as easy as it sounds, these two elements are the foundation of every treatment plan. Doctors know that changes in lifestyle habits can head off many syndrome X conditions before they gain a hold on your body, so it makes good sense to use them to end the progression of damage as well. Wellness is really about establishing lifestyle habits you can live with for a lifetime and that can carry you through a long life. Encourage other family members to develop more healthy habits too. Change is always easier if there are others involved.

Regular medical care, including checkups for blood sugar and lipid levels, high blood pressure, and, if you have diabetes or hypertension, proteins in the urine that could signal early kidney disease should also be a part of your new lifestyle. If your doctor has prescribed medication, take it as directed. If you notice new signs or symptoms, contact your doctor to have them evaluated. In the end, your health is your responsibility—for the best results, you must be an active participant in safeguarding and caring for it.

What progress are researchers making to determine why syndrome X develops?

Researchers are making tremendous progress in their understanding of potential genetic factors that contribute to insulin resistance and obesity. Research centers across the nation are exploring various aspects of diabetes, obesity, and genetics as they apply to the conditions of syndrome X. Some studies are examining the concept of the thrifty gene theory, attempting to unravel the mysteries of why this ancient survival mechanism has stayed "on" despite significant changes in the environment that make it now more of a hazard than a help. Once researchers fully understand the involvement of insulin resistance and diabetes, they will be able to look at other syndrome X conditions such as dyslipidemia and PCOS and develop more effective treatments.

What progress are researchers making to develop new treatments for syndrome X?

Each new discovery about a potential cause for a syndrome X condition leads to new treatments. Some approaches target prevention. Others target treatment, such as medications.

MEDICATIONS

The newest drugs to hit the market to show great promise in treating type 2 diabetes, PCOS, and other presentations of insulin resistance are the insulin-sensitizing drugs. These drugs are becoming more sophisticated as researchers learn how to tailor their effects to focus on particular aspects of cell activities. New classes of drugs act to improve insulin resistance in different ways, often with fewer side effects.

A great deal of attention is also being focused on identifying and synthesizing substances found naturally in the body that may influence obesity and insulin resistance. One such substance is the hormone leptin, which is released by fat cells. Researchers are continuing to study leptin and its role in appetite. It or substances like it could be the key that turns on and off a person's desire to eat.

THE ROLE OF GENES

Researchers studying obesity have identified several "fat" genes that, when damaged, cause obesity to develop. These studies just involve laboratory animals at this point. Other researchers are working to identify the genes that produce and regulate insulin. This could lead to new ways to treat both obesity and diabetes, and would likely reveal a new understanding of how hypertension, dyslipidemia, and other forms of heart disease develop and progress. Gene therapy could be used to treat virtually any condition with a hereditary component, with the prospect of eliminating the disease entirely. Such a manipulation could eventually occur before the condition even develops.

BIOTECHNOLOGY

Many people view biotechnology as a thing of the future—the distant future. This is not so. Biotechnology (the process of using knowledge to manipulate nature) has been a part of everyday life since ancient societies planted certain crops next to each other so they could cross-pollinate and produce stronger, healthier plants. Today, biotechnology touches nearly every aspect of modern life, from stonewashed denim jeans to bottled soda. Manufacturers use synthesized enzymes to produce these and dozens of other everyday products. But by far the most significant developments of biotechnology are in medicine.

The most obvious example of this is antibiotics. In a quantum leap from their humble origins on a moldy piece of bread, most antibiotics today are developed in laboratories, the products of careful manipulations of cells and even molecules to create agents that can target and kill specific bacteria. Scientists believe the antibiotics of the future will no longer attack bacteria but will alter cells in the body to make them resistant to the bacteria. Ultimately, many researchers believe, nearly all medications could function this way. The newest insulin-sensitizing drugs are not so far removed from this futuristic scenario, in that they specifically target cell insulin receptors. Other potential applications for bioengineered drugs are hormones such as leptin, which could be synthesized if they prove effective in treating health problems such as diabetes and insulin resistance. Bioengineered drugs might also be useful in fighting dyslipidemia and reducing the fatty plaque buildups that occur inside the arteries when blood lipid levels remain too high.

LIFESTYLE

As researchers move closer to understanding the genetic components of insulin resistance and diabetes, they are gaining new knowledge about how environment and behavior influence the body in carrying out its genetic predispositions. They are studying what effects a high-fat diet has on dyslipidemia and cardiovascular disease, for example, when such a predisposition exists and when it does not. Researchers are also continuing to learn more about the many different blood lipids, and to distinguish their roles in health as well as in disease.

Evidence supporting the integral role of lifestyle habits is so compelling that a number of health organizations are targeting lifestyle changes as an approach to preventing the onset of type 2 diabetes and hypertension. These prevention initiatives, as they are often called, emphasize extensive education and outreach efforts to get information to people who are at risk for developing these conditions.

Are there other conditions that could be part of syndrome X?

It is likely that there are other health problems linked to syndrome X. High homocysteine levels and certain specific lipid abnormalities other than those already known to be present with syndrome X dyslipidemia may be related.

These conditions often appear in people who have insulin resistance, diabetes, or other syndrome X conditions.

Homocysteine is a natural waste product your body makes when it metabolizes protein. Most people have enzymes in their bodies that immediately mobilize to neutralize homocysteine, keeping its level in your body low. In some people, this reaction is a bit sluggish and homocysteine accumulates in the bloodstream. High homocysteine levels are an indicator of early, and often serious, heart disease. A diet high in B vitamins, especially folic acid, seems to stimulate the enzymes that are slow to react, restoring them to near normal function. Foods high in folic acid include broccoli, cauliflower, peas, spinach, and tofu (a soybean product). Also, many packaged foods such as breakfast cereals and even snack crackers contain added folic acid.

This relationship between homocysteine levels and folic acid raises the possibility that vitamins and minerals may influence other conditions of syndrome X. This is an exciting direction of research, because vitamin therapy would be inexpensive and easy. Other vitamin relationships being examined include vitamin E and heart disease, and vitamin C and immune disorders (including type 1 diabetes). Pinning down these kinds of connections could greatly expand the whole notion of prevention through diet.

Does it look likely that researchers will figure out how to "break the chain" of syndrome X?

Researchers are quite optimistic that they will soon understand precisely how insulin resistance links the conditions of syndrome X. While they know there is a significant correlation between obesity and insulin resistance and subsequent health problems with syndrome X conditions, they do not know for sure what mechanisms allow this correlation to develop into a disease state. Understanding these connections seems to be the key to understanding syndrome X and its conditions.

Can I expect a cure for diabetes in my lifetime?

Researchers are very close to unlocking the secrets of how insulin works, leading to great hope that diabetes will be as much a disease of the past in the United States as is smallpox by the time today's youngsters become adults. The Diabetes Prevention Trial for Type 1 Diabetes might be the first successful attempt to prevent type 1 diabetes. Other possibilities discussed earlier, such as bioengineered drugs, may also prove to be permanent cures for diabetes in the near future (the next 10 to 20 years). And there is compelling evidence that type 2 diabetes in particular appears to be preventable, if intervention occurs early enough to avoid obesity.

Even if a cure—defined as permanently eliminating the condition so treatment is no longer necessary—is a bit further down the research road, effective long-term treatments are just around the corner. We might eventually view treatment with insulin-sensitizing drugs in the same way we do treating hypothyroidism with thyroid supplements—just the minor inconvenience of taking a pill. Though this is not a cure in the traditional sense, it does remove symptoms of disease and restore health as long as the medication is taken. This could subsequently reduce the risk for developing complications or other conditions within the syndrome X constellation.

If researchers discover a cure for insulin resistance and diabetes, will it be a cure for syndrome X as well?

The underlying factor linking the conditions of syndrome X seems to be insulin resistance. In fact, insulin resistance could be thought of as the precursor to all of the features of syndrome X, including type 2 diabetes. So it seems logical that finding a cure for insulin resistance, or at least a treatment that could permanently suppress signs and symptoms, would also be a cure for syndrome X.

How close are researchers to figuring out how to prevent heart disease?

With certain types of heart disease, researchers are closing in on prevention. We know, for instance, that exercise, a healthy diet, and not smoking will prevent a lot of heart disease. However, we also know that some people develop heart disease despite taking all the right measures to prevent it. This probably speaks to a genetic factor of some sort, or risks that as yet remain unknown. It also tells us that not all heart disease is associated with insulin resistance or diabetes—at least as far as current research supports. Other variables may be involved in some situations. We do not fully understand, for example, why estrogen apparently fails to protect premenopausal women who have diabetes from heart disease as it does in women who do not have diabetes. Nor do we understand how a person with normal blood lipid levels can have a heart attack after which examination reveals seriously occluded coronary arteries. Though we know correlations exist between certain factors, we do not fully understand how they influence the development of disease.

How does heart disease research affect syndrome X treatment?

Because syndrome X is a significant risk factor for serious or advanced heart disease, there is much research focused on identifying the connections. Some researchers believe all heart disease has some sort of insulin-resistance connection, though there is not yet conclusive evidence to support this. Other researchers believe that while insulin resistance sets the stage for heart disease, once heart disease begins, it runs its own course. After that point, it does not matter what set it up—what matters is heading it off. In this respect, any treatment that targets the symptoms of advanced heart disease (such as serious cardiovascular disease and damage to the heart muscle itself) has relevance for all heart disease regardless of the factors that precipitated its development.

What research is going on specifically regarding syndrome X?

Most research targets the collective symptoms of the conditions, looking for explanations for how the conditions are linked and what happens if you break the link by treating the insulin resistance. This is a complex area of research, because we know that while treating insulin resistance reduces the risk for developing complications and additional conditions, there is as yet no evidence that treating the insulin resistance can reverse heart disease. The elements are very intertwined. Is it obesity that sets the stage for diabetes and hypertension, or insulin resistance? Researchers do not yet know.

How do I stay informed about new discoveries?

As we move deeper into a technology-driven culture, acquiring information will become less significant an issue than separating hope from healing. The Internet has opened wide the doors to almost too much information. Many reputable organizations have established websites that provide up-to-the-minute reports on new technologies and new treatments. Several government organizations sponsor research studies and report on new findings, such as the National Institutes of Health (NIH). Local and national organizations such as the American Heart Association, the American Diabetes Association, and the National Kidney Foundation report on new research. These organizations also typically assess the practicality of new treatment approaches. Other reputable health organizations offer similar information. The "Resources" section at the end of this book provides a listing to get you started.

A word of caution about reports of new discoveries is also in order here, however. Be wary of reports that seem too good to be true, or that are testimonials from people who have tried the discovery and found it to work wonders. Reputable research uses scientific, objective methods to study and report findings. Testimonials and personal experience are not objective and may not be reliable. Unfortunately, they are often the hallmark of disreputable efforts to sell products of questionable effectiveness. They may suggest that conventional researchers have closed their eyes to the amazing success of what surely is the most miraculous medical discovery of the century. This should be a huge red flag. Legitimate research does not rely on hyperbole. It presents the good and the bad, the helpful and the hazardous. We cannot say it enough: If it sounds too good to be true, it probably is. Occasionally the medical community does become excited about a breakthrough in prevention, diagnosis, or treatment. When this happens, you will be able to find numerous research studies all reporting the same findings.

How can I be sure my doctor is staying informed about new treatment approaches and options?

So much new information is becoming available on almost a daily basis that it is impossible for everyone to keep up with everything. Doctors who specialize in treating syndrome X conditions are most likely to be current regarding prevention and treatment options. Some divisions among specialties still challenge the dissemination of new information. For example, many doctors who treat patients with diabetes and heart disease do not usually treat women who have PCOS. Women with PCOS often receive care from gynecologists or fertility experts. As doctors are learning more about the interrelationships that exist among the various conditions of syndrome X, they are revising the way they think about and treat their patients who present with symptoms of just one (like PCOS).

Ask your doctor what he or she keeps up with in the areas of prevention and treatment for syndrome X conditions. This will give you a better sense for how to focus your own efforts to keep current. Knowing that you are interested in the latest information may encourage your doctor to take notice when relevant material appears in professional journals and other sources. Your doctor might also be able to direct you to reliable resources, so you can better keep up with what is new. Your doctor can then further explore approaches and techniques that might benefit you in your unique and specific circumstances. Most doctor-patient relationships function best when they are partnerships.

How do I know if a new treatment will help me?

This is really more of a challenge than finding information about new treatments. Despite the similarities that link the conditions of syndrome X, treatment is a very customized process. What works for some people does not work for others. The best place to start is with a knowledgeable physician. Hopefully this is the doctor who is guiding your care, though sometimes it is necessary to seek a specialist through a reputable source such as a professional organization or a clinic affiliated with a research center. Often you can contact a physician whose name appears in reports about new discoveries. This doctor can either provide you with additional information or refer you to someone who can. While many doctors who become involved in research projects also see patients, some do not.

Learn as much as you can about the new treatment before you discuss it with the doctor (whether you plan to contact your regular doctor or a new specialist). This gives you a base from which to ask informed questions, and from which to understand the responses. Not every treatment will work for every patient who has similar symptoms. Whether a new treatment will work for *you* may not be apparent before you try it. On the flip side, there may be characteristics of your circumstances that suggest a new treatment will not work for you. In either case, it helps if you know enough about both your health conditions and the new treatment to accept or reject the doctor's responses. Doctors, too, have their biases about treatment approaches. It is important to understand why your doctor supports or rejects a treatment that interests you.

What do I do if a new treatment sounds promising but my doctor doesn't want to try it?

Decisions about your health care ultimately reside with you. Your relationship with your doctor should be such that you can ask questions and receive useful answers. Your mutual respect should be motivated by a shared concern for your health. Your doctor may have good reasons for rejecting a new treatment. It could be that the studies are not complete, or the findings are inconsistent with the findings of other studies in the same area. It could be that the risks of the prospective treatment outweigh the potential benefits for all but a certain few patients. It is not always clear, especially in consumer-oriented health information, what kinds of patients were involved in the research study. Sometimes the study has not yet involved patients but has yielded exciting results in a laboratory environment.

Discuss your interest in the new treatment with the doctor who is guiding your care for your syndrome X conditions. If he or she remains resistant, see a different specialist for a second opinion. You can ask your regular doctor to recommend someone, if you are comfortable in doing this. (Patients have far more anxiety about this than do doctors. Doctors are quite used to consultations and second opinions, and do not consider requests for them as any kind of a personal affront.) Be sure the specialist you see is involved in the area of treatment that interests you. A fertility expert who treats many women with PCOS is likely to give a more informed consultation than is a general gynecologist who occasionally sees someone with the condition, for example. Likewise, an internist who sees patients who have conditions across a broad spectrum of diabetes, hypertension, dyslipidemia, and even kidney disease is likely to have more interest in and knowledge of syndrome X treatment approaches than is a cardiologist who sees mostly patients in the later stages of heart disease.

If the second specialist is willing to try the new treatment, be sure he or she has your complete medical record and understands what approaches you have tried so far. Be sure, too, that you have realistic expectations about the new treatment. At this point in time, while many treatments show great promise, there are no cures for the conditions of syndrome X. Is this new treatment considered experimental? If so, be sure your health insurance will pay for it. If you receive this new treatment, are you actually participating in clinical trials to see how well it works in "real life" situations? This is not necessarily a bad thing, just something you should thoroughly understand in terms of risks and benefits before you move forward. Such participation requires informed consent on your part, so be especially clear about what happens if something goes wrong or the treatment causes more health problems than you already have.

Remember that all new treatments generate great excitement within the medical community when they appear to have the potential to make significant changes in patient health. Not all of this potential becomes reality. Usually, by the time a treatment (including a medication) is approved for use with a particular condition, it has been through exhaustive testing. This does not mean, however, that it is 100% safe or foolproof. Often as a drug or treatment receives widespread use, new findings crop up. Some are positive, some are adverse. If you begin a treatment that is new for your condition, keep up on your reading with the same diligence you had when you first discovered the information. This is one way to find out what, if any, additional findings are being reported as more patients try the treatment.

How do I keep myself as healthy as possible?

The best way to stay healthy is to take care of yourself. Eat nutritiously, stay active, and get regular checkups from your doctor. Stay informed about new developments in prevention and treatment. Do not focus solely on your health conditions, though. Engage yourself in activities that you enjoy, and find ways to relax.

~

Resources and Additional Information

With new information surfacing at an astounding rate, the Internet is your best resource for keeping up with what is new. But before you start web-surfing, we have a note of caution. There is much (some people say too much) information available on the Internet. Some of it is reliable, coming from trusted sources that only report the findings and results of reputable, scientific studies. These sources are often national organizations or websites sponsored by universities and research centers. Unfortunately, there is also a vast amount of misinformation available on the Internet. Unlike most print publications, which typically verify documentation and sources for their articles, the Internet has few controls. Anyone can post just about anything.

Be wary of websites that present personal experiences. Such a site is usually the product of an individual who has a particular medical condition (or interest in it), a person who probably has no medical training. He or she reports what has been of personal interest or effectiveness, generally without independent corroboration or substantiation. People who create their own websites also obtain information from other websites. As a result, erroneous information can spread through Internet websites faster than dandelions invade neighborhood lawns.

If you do not have access to the Internet at home or at

work, spend an afternoon at the public library. Most have computers with Internet access that are available at no charge to library card holders. Some libraries impose time limits during peak hours, so it is a good idea to check with yours before planning to spend the day researching the health topics that interest you. Many libraries also allow you to print materials from the Internet, though some charge a small fee for doing so. The library is also a good place to peruse medical journals for the latest research findings and treatment information. Some medical journals are available online (on the Internet) as well, though may require you to register or subscribe to obtain in-depth information.

The following websites offer information about the conditions of syndrome X. All offer free access unless otherwise noted.

American Diabetes Association
www.diabetes.org
Provides information on the latest research studies and treatments, as well as general information about diabetes, nutrition, and exercise. Written for consumers.

American Heart Association
www.amhrt.org
This website provides comprehensive information about all aspects of heart disease, including hypertension, dyslipidemia, coronary artery disease, and cerebral artery disease. It offers suggestions for establishing healthy lifestyle habits to help prevent heart disease.

Center for PCOS
www.centerforpcos.bsd.uchicago.edu
The University of Chicago's Center for PCOS sponsors research and educational efforts about polycystic ovarian syndrome. The website provides information about the latest research studies and new treatment approaches.

Mayo Clinic Health Oasis

www.mayohealth.org

This website, sponsored by the Mayo Clinic, offers comprehensive information about all kinds of health topics. Many sections also provide excellent links to additional resources.

Medscape

www.medscape.com

This website requires free registration. It provides a broad range of health information and clinical articles from various sources.

National Diabetes Education Initiative

www.ndei.org

This website features articles and updates to educate doctors about a wide range of topics related to diabetes.

National Diabetes Information Clearinghouse

www.niddk.nih.gov

The National Diabetes Information Clearinghouse is part of the National Institutes of Health. This website reports on new research findings and provides a variety of statistics.

National Institutes of Health

www.nih.gov/icd/

This webpage lists links for the websites of the 25 separate institutes and centers that comprise the National Institutes of Health, including The National Heart, Lung, and Blood Institute (NHLBI); the National Institute of Diabetes and Digestive and Kidney Diseases (NIDDK); the National Center for Complementary and Alternative Medicine (NCCAM); and the National Library of Medicine (NLM).

Partnership for Healthy Weight Management

www.consumer.gov/weightloss/

This site is sponsored by the federal government to educate

consumers about what to expect from weight-loss products and programs. It provides a body mass index (BMI) chart and information about weight control and choosing an appropriate weight-loss program.

Stanford University School of Medicine
www.syndromex.stanford.edu
This website is sponsored by the Stanford University School of Medicine General Clinic Research Center. The site follows ongoing syndrome X studies and the work of syndrome X researcher Dr. Gerald Reavens.

Index